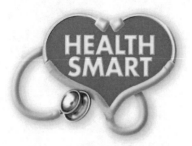

HOSPITAL HANDBOOK

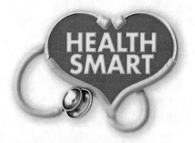

HOSPITAL HANDBOOK

Joseph Sacco, M.D.

ALPHA

A member of Penguin Group (USA) Inc.

For Mimi, without whom this book—and many other good things—would never have happened, and for Rosie and Sarah.

International Standard Book Number: 1-59257-075-5
Library of Congress Catalog Card Number: 2003106906

05 04 03   8 7 6 5 4 3 2 1

Interpretation of the printing code: The rightmost number of the first series of numbers is the year of the book's printing; the rightmost number of the second series of numbers is the number of the book's printing. For example, a printing code of 03-1 shows that the first printing occurred in 2003.

Printed in the United States of America

Contents

Introduction

I began writing this book after my mother had a heart attack in the fall of 2001. I had been working in a hospital in the South Bronx for almost a decade, providing inpatient medical care for thousands of people. I had even cared for my father at home when he was dying from lung cancer, but the passage of years had tempered my sensitivity to the concerns of my patients and their families. Then my mother was admitted to the cardiac care unit at Lenox Hill Hospital on Manhattan's Upper East Side. Suddenly, I was asking the same anxious questions I had been hearing for years. Was she going to be okay? Was she getting the right treatments and medications? Who was her head doctor? Should I talk to her cardiologist or her pulmonary specialist about her condition? Would she be able to go home when she got better, or would she need rehab? What about help with cooking, shopping, and cleaning?

I was lucky. My experience as a doctor helped me to get my questions answered because I was already aware of which questions to ask. I had a solid understanding of my mother's illness and treatment, the risks associated with the cardiac care unit (CCU), who to go to for information, when to make a fuss (as well as how to talk to doctors without treading on their notoriously fragile egos), and dozens of other details about her care.

Today, she's back in her apartment on the East Side, cooking, cleaning, and shopping, as well as seeing friends, going to movies, and volunteering at a nearby elementary school, just like she did before she became ill. The credit for her recovery goes to the doctors and nurses at Lenox Hill for the fantastic job they did, and to my mother for her fortitude and determination to get better. Still, my advocacy helped make sure that her hospital stay was as short and safe as possible, and that she got out in far better shape than when she went in.

The Importance of Communication

One of the ways you'll be able to make the most of your hospital stay is by understanding what your doctor is saying. Chapter 16 summarizes common medical terms, and Appendix A lists medical terminology and slang. Acronyms such as CCU (cardiac care unit) are very common in the medical world and are sprinkled liberally throughout this book, enabling you to learn the lingo as you read. If a term is in italics, you can quickly look up the word in the glossary at the back of the book.

Unfortunately, most people who are confronted by a hospital stay do not have the benefit of this knowledge, and neither do their relatives. Although I have long familiarity with the nuts and bolts of hospitals, it was not until my mother's heart attack that I began to understand what the experience *feels* like, or, at least, how it feels to have a hospitalized loved one.

If I, a *hospitalist* (a specialist in the care of hospitalized patients), was feeling adrift, my patients, I imagined, must be completely lost. What they needed was what I already had: a sound base of information about the entire hospital experience, from the 15-hour wait in the emergency room to delivery by wheelchair outside the main entrance for the car ride home. So I decided to put it all down on paper: twenty years of accumulated knowledge about doctors, nurses, medications, operating rooms, x-rays, blood tests, the whole gamut ... a handbook to being in the hospital.

It is my hope that by providing a few fundamentals on health and illness, a solid description of the hospital experience, and the inside track on how to advocate for yourself (or your loved one) in the medical bureaucracy, you will not only reap the maximum benefit from a hospital stay, but also learn how to work with your doctor or health-care provider to live a longer and healthier life.

A Few Hospital Statistics

In 1999, 32,100,000 Americans were admitted to the hospital, for a total of 160,100,000 days. That's just over one in ten American men, women, and children, each of whom spent an average of five days in the hospital[1].

Who are all these people, and why are they in the hospital? Good question. The elderly (those over 65), comprising 12 percent of the population in the 2000 census (35 million people), make up the single largest group of hospital patients. In 1999, they accounted for 12,683,000 admissions, or 40 percent of the total. Heart disease, including heart attack, angina, abnormal heart rhythm (*arrhythmia*), and heart failure, is the most common cause for elderly people to be admitted, comprising almost 25 percent (2.889 million) of cases[1].

The following table lists the other top reasons elderly people are admitted.

Ten Leading Causes of Hospital Admission (in Descending Order), Age 65 and Over (1999)

Diagnosis	Hospitalizations (Annually, 1999)	Rate per 10,000 Population
Heart disease (including heart attack, abnormal heartbeat, and heart failure)	2,889,000	843.7
Pneumonia	810,000	236.5
Cancer (including colon, rectum, and lung)	729,000	212.8
Cerebrovascular disease (including stroke)	704,000	205.5
Fractures	531,000	155.2
Chronic bronchitis	369,000	107.8
Joint disease (including arthritis)	303,000	88.6

continues

Ten Leading Causes of Hospital Admission (in Descending Order), Age 65 and Over (1999) *continued*

Diagnosis	Hospitalizations (Annually, 1999)	Rate per 10,000 Population
Dehydration	247,000	72.2
Sepsis (blood infection)	241,000	70.5
Mental illness	212,000	62

From: 1999 National Hospital Discharge Survey, Centers for Disease Control and Prevention, U.S. Department of Health and Human Services.

What about the other 60 percent of admissions? These are accounted for by people under 65. Almost 7 million people between 45 and 64 were admitted to the hospital in 1999, 10 million between 14 and 44, and 2.5 million under 15. The reasons? Heart disease and stroke—the predominant reasons for admission in the elderly—remain the primary reasons for admittance in those 45 to 64, while mental illness, trauma, and *acute* problems such as appendicitis, colitis, and kidney stones are the more common causes in those 44 and under (doctors refer to illnesses of recent onset as *acute;* nonmedical people use the term to mean that an illness is of great severity).

The following tables list the most common causes of admission for people in the age groups of 15 to 44 and 45 to 64[1].

Ages 15 to 44

Diagnosis	Number of Admissions	Rate per 10,000 Population
Mental disorders (including psychoses and alcohol dependence)	1,167,000	95.6
Injury and poisoning (including fractures)	787,000	64.5
Digestive disorders (including appendicitis, colitis, diverticula, and gallstones)	747,000	61.2
Genitourinary disorders (including kidney stones)	568,000	46.6

Diagnosis	Number of Admissions	Rate per 10,000 Population
Complications of pregnancy and childbirth	491,000	40.3
Respiratory disease (including pneumonia, asthma, and bronchitis)	430,000	35.3
Circulatory disease (including heart disease and stroke)	417,000	34.2
Musculoskeletal disorders (including arthritis and intervertebral disc disease)	326,000	26.7
Neoplasms (including malignant and benign)	283,000	23.2
Endocrine/metabolic disorders (including diabetes and dehydration)	264,000	26.1

Ages 45 to 64

Diagnosis	Number of Admissions	Rate per 10,000 Population
Circulatory disease (including heart disease and stroke)	1,797,000	304.5
Digestive disorders (including appendicitis, colitis, diverticula, and gallstones)	830,000	140.6
Respiratory disease (including pneumonia, asthma, and bronchitis)	686,000	116.3
Neoplasms (including malignant and benign)	486,000	95.8
Injury and poisoning (including fractures)	526,000	89.1
Mental disorders (including psychoses and alcohol dependence)	486,000	82.1

continues

Ages 45 to 64 *continued*

Diagnosis	Number of Admissions	Rate per 10,000 Population
Musculoskeletal disorders (including arthritis and intervertebral disc disease)	481,000	81.6
Genitourinary disorders (including kidney stones)	428,000	72.6
Endocrine/metabolic disorders (including Diabetes and Dehydration)	351,000	59.5
Skin disease (including skin infections and abscesses)	134,000	22.6

A more accurate picture of who's in the hospital, however, requires looking not only at which diseases result in admission, but why people get sick to start with. For example, does diet influence hospitalization? Does it make a difference whether people smoke or exercise regularly? What about heredity and gender? And who spends more time in the hospital, people who are overweight, or those who, medically speaking, are a healthier weight?

Many factors influence illness, and lifestyle factors such as smoking, diet, weight, and exercise are especially important. The primary goal of *HealthSmart Hospital Handbook* is to maximize the benefits and reduce the risks of your hospital stay. Even better would be to keep you *out* of the hospital to start with.

Does the fact that lifestyle is so important to the prevention of disease mean that *people* are the cause of illness? No! People are the victims, not the cause, of illness. There might be room for improvement in the health habits of Americans, but no one asks to get sick. Further, many people suffer from "preventable" conditions despite following all the rules. They lose weight, stop smoking, exercise more, and improve their diets and still get cancer, respiratory illness, and heart disease.

Illness, in other words, happens. Most of us, at one point or another, young or old, skinny or overweight, are going to wind up in the hospital. So read on, and you will learn all you need to know after you're there.

Other Influences on Your Hospital Stay

Illness happens, and doctors are entrusted to heal the sick. Yet many other factors will influence your hospital stay, social, political, and financial undercurrents that have profoundly changed the way modern medicine is practiced. These factors, and the chapters covering them, include the following:

+ Medical errors, and nosocomial (hospital-caused) and iatrogenic (doctor-caused) illness (Chapters 3, 17, and 18).
+ Managed care and the crisis of the underinsured and uninsured (Chapter 3).
+ Increased regulatory and paperwork requirements and a critical shortage of nurses (Chapter 3).
+ Medical malpractice and its influence on medical practice and the availability of services (Chapter 3 and 20).
+ A dramatically altered relationship between doctor and patient (Chapter 7).
+ Greatly expanded patients' rights (Chapter 5).
+ A new focus on pain management (Chapter 14).
+ A humanistic, rather than disease-oriented approach to care at the end-of-life (Chapter 19).

In Medicine, Knowledge Is Power

Knowledge is essential to effective patient advocacy. Studies have shown that patients who feel that they have actively participated in a treatment plan are more likely to feel satisfied with their care and to comply with the agreed upon plan of treatment[2]. This translates into less time in the hospital, less exposure to hospital-borne dangers, faster recovery, and a smaller likelihood that relapse will put them right back where they started. Likewise, the friend, relative, or loved one of a patient who is unable to advocate for him- or herself (for example, someone who is critically ill, unconscious, or on a respirator) will be far more able to effectively direct doctors and nurses from an informed base of knowledge.

If someone you care about is in the hospital, ask the same questions, seek the same information, and insist on the same high-quality care as you would for yourself. Strong and caring advocacy can enormously improve their hospital experience, which is a central goal of *HealthSmart Hospital Handbook*.

So be sure to pay close attention to the "Good questions and suggestions for your doctor concerning …" sections at the end of each chapter. They will help you gather the information you need for this advocacy—and inform your doctor of your preferences.

Acknowledgments

With my thanks and gratitude to Gary Goldstein, Nancy Lewis, Molly Schaller, Christy Wagner, and Sherry Wulkan for their hard work, excellent advice, and tireless assistance in creating the *HealthSmart Hospital Handbook*.

Chapter 1

Need to Go to the Hospital? Perhaps You Can Stay Home!

Let's say you've got a nasty cold, and after a week of a hacking cough you developed a high fever, drenching sweats, and chills. Today, you visited your doctor, and the news wasn't good. The doctor listened to your chest with a stethoscope, frowned, and told you have pneumonia and need to be admitted to the hospital for intravenous antibiotics.

What now? Do you really have to go to the hospital? Are there *any* alternatives?

Yes. There are many alternatives to hospitalization. More and more, conditions once felt to require in-hospital care are now being managed at home or in "sub-acute" settings such as nursing homes or rehab centers. Further, many people who do need to be admitted are being discharged early, with the lion's share of treatment being completed at home. Home health care, in which preventive, diagnostic, and curative services are delivered by doctors, nurses, and other health-care professionals in peoples' houses (or by the patients themselves after appropriate training) is a fast growing segment of the health-care industry with many benefits for patients[1].

How can you take advantage of these services? This chapter will explore home health care, so that even when you must go to the hospital, the "hospital" you go to will be in the comfort of your own home.

But first, let's re-examine an important question: Does your condition really merit in-hospital care? And are there other factors that influence the decision to admit?

Reasons for Admission: More Than Just Sickness

Doctors admit people for many reasons, not all of which have to do with the need to be in the hospital. Many who report to emergency rooms have conditions that might easily be managed at home, but, lacking a primary care doctor who can monitor their progress, wind up being admitted to assure the success of therapy. Others are admitted to expedite a diagnostic work-up that could be completed on an outpatient basis. Or a patient might have other medical problems that make at-home management risky. An otherwise healthy young woman with mild pneumonia and a good primary care doctor, for example, might be sent home, while the same patient with a history of asthma might be admitted because of the possibility she might start wheezing and need closely supervised care.

What does all of this mean for you? For one, having a primary care doctor means being able to assure the doctor in the emergency room that follow-up will not be a problem. You can even ask the ER doctor to call your primary care doctor and establish a plan of outpatient care over the phone. Next, whether you are in the emergency room or your doctor's office, you can avoid being admitted to the hospital for testing such as CAT scans or MRIs by offering to do some of the footwork needed to get these tests done as an outpatient yourself. Doctors and their office staff have been deluged by paperwork in the last decade, and usually have to fill out a handful of forms and await insurance company approval before your appointments for testing can be made. Offer to help! Get on the phone and push your insurance company to approve the tests you need. If you are informed about your condition, you'll be all the more able to convey the urgency of your condition. You and your doctor are a team not only when it comes to agreeing on a treatment plan, but also in cutting through the maze of bureaucracy to get things done.

If you a have chronic illness such as asthma, get regular care, take your medications, and keep it under control to help avoid admission. The young woman with asthma is much less likely to be admitted for pneumonia if she diligently uses prescribed asthma medications, doesn't smoke, hasn't had an asthma attack in years, and can readily get an appointment with her primary care doctor. Not only does controlling chronic illness make it less likely that an acute illness will cause trouble (remember, "acute" refers to a problem of recent onset), but it is also a good indication that the affected individual will reliably take medications and attend follow-up.

These are common sense examples of ways you can assist your doctor—the doctor in the emergency room or your primary care doctor—in making the decision to treat you at home rather than admitting you to the hospital.

And if you still need treatment, such as intravenous therapy or wound care, that is traditionally thought of as hospital-based?

The Hospital-at-Home Options

As discussed, home health care can perform many of the tasks once available only in the hospital. This gives you the option to stay at home even when the "hospital" is deemed necessary. Services available are described in the sections that follow.

Intravenous Therapy

Intravenous catheters allow fluids and medications to be administered directly into the blood stream. Home health care makes home IV therapy possible. Practically speaking, though, conditions worth treating in this fashion are those requiring several weeks, or even months, of medication. Home IV therapy typically uses *central lines*, catheters that are threaded into the major vessels of the abdomen or chest, and these are not without complications.

There are several types of central lines; those used at home include the *PICC* (*peripherally inserted central catheter*), *Hickman*, and *Portacath*. PICC lines are usually inserted into the vein in the crook of the elbow and are placed under local anesthesia; both the Hickman and Portacath are placed under general anesthesia in the upper chest and risk collapse of the lung during insertion (several inches of catheter extend outside the chest with the Hickman; the Portacath is buried completely under the skin).

Apria Healthcare, a medical supply company, has an informative web page about central lines at www.apria.com. Click the Resources tab and select FAQs, then select Infusion Therapy—General or Infusion Therapy—Safety. (See Chapter 17 for more information on dangers related to central lines.)

Home IVs can be used to give just about any medication or fluid that is given in the hospital, including *saline* (plain, ordinary salt water used to treat dehydration or to maintain hydration in people who are unable to eat or drink), pain medications, nutrients for people with gastrointestinal disorders that interfere with eating or who need extra nutrients during or after prolonged illness (*parenteral nutrition*), blood transfusion, heart medications, and others.

Infusion catheters can also be placed under the skin (*subcutaneously*), a simple and common method for providing pain medication to the terminally ill, and next to the spine (*epidural*), a technique also useful in pain management.

Physical and Occupational Therapy

People recovering from a stroke, amputation, prolonged immobilization after orthopedic surgery or a fracture, burns, head trauma, and other conditions might need help in recovering physical function. Physical therapists help speed the recovery of *motor skills* such as walking and moving from sitting to standing; occupational therapists focus on *activities of daily living* (ADLs) such as using utensils, going to the toilet, and getting dressed.

Podiatry

Medical illness can result in some very unpleasant foot problems. Reduction of blood flow from narrowed arteries and reduced sensation from nerve damage (*neuropathy*) in diabetics, for example, is a leading cause of gangrene and amputation. Podiatrists help diabetics and others with foot problems keep their feet clean and dry, attend to nail care, corns, and bunions, and provide advice on footwear that will help prevent foot injury.

Dietary Services

Many people—diabetics provide another good example—have medical conditions that require dietary therapy. A nutritionist, visiting at home, can help with meal planning and go through refrigerators and cupboards to suggest needed changes.

Nursing

Without nurses, home care would come to nothing. Nurses do *everything*, from infusion therapy and wound care to hospice services for the terminally ill. More on nursing care in Chapter 7 and more on hospice in Chapter 19.

Laboratory Testing

Need a blood test, but too sick to get out of bed? The medications used to treat blood clots, for example, need to be monitored regularly to assure that blood thinning is just right. Too much, and you might bleed, too little, and the clot might spread. Never fear! A lab technician will go to your house, draw your blood, and report the results to your doctor, a perfect example of the coordinated, multidisciplinary services available through home health care.

Treatment of Blood Clots

Blood clots (*deep venous thrombosis*, DVT) cause pain and swelling in the veins of the leg. Untreated, they can travel to the lungs, causing severe shortness of breath and death (*pulmonary embolus*). Heparin, an injectable blood thinner (*anticoagulant*), and Coumadin (*warfarin*), an oral anticoagulant, are used to dissolve the clot.

Home Attendant and Home Health Aide Services

Twenty-four-hour-a-day, seven-day-a-week home care might be necessary for people who live alone and are unable to care for themselves. Elderly people who suffer a stroke or the memory and intellectual losses associated with dementia are good candidates for 24-hour home care. *Home attendants* help people with cooking, cleaning, and shopping, accompany their charges to doctor's appointments, and assist with light personal care such as bathing. *Home health aides,* who have more training, emphasize feeding, bathing, changing diapers, and other personal care needs. Both are formally trained and certified, and neither is permitted to administer medications. But take note! Most insurance agencies, including Medicare, will not pay for custodial services such as a home attendant or home health aide unless a skilled need, such as nursing, is also required.

At Home *After* Hospital Services

Admittedly, many home-hospital services begin after people are discharged from the hospital. Serious infections, for example, usually require at least some period in the hospital for initial treatment, with the switch to home health care when the condition has been stabilized. Likewise, surgery *cannot* be done at home. Same-day surgery centers, which conduct surgery in the morning and send people home in the afternoon, *depend* on home health services. Likewise, the trend to shorter and shorter hospital stays has made home health services a must for people who continue to need close follow-up and care after discharge.

Do You Qualify for Home Care?

Talk with your doctor, making it clear that you prefer a hospital-at-home to the more customary form of hospital admission. If you do require admission, insist on the earliest possible discharge to home care. By all accounts, you will get better quicker, have fewer costs, and have less exposure to the risks associated with the hospital.

Insurance Coverage of Home Health-Care Services

Medicare, Medicaid, and private insurers are the major financiers of home health care. Home health care is cheaper than in-hospital care, making it an attractive alternative for both publicly and privately financed insurance. The following sections detail some of the home health-care services available through these insurers.

Medicare

To be eligible for home care financed by Medicare, you must already be a Medicare beneficiary; care must include skilled nursing, physical, speech, or occupational therapy; and you must be homebound. (*Skilled nursing* is that which can only be performed safely and properly by a registered nurse or licensed practical nurse, such as wound care or IV infusions.) Medicare will also pay for a home health aide, but once skilled care is no longer required, this service is not covered. Medicare also pays for a social worker, medical supplies such as wound dressings and an oxygen tank (minus a 20 percent co-payment), but not for prescription drugs or a home attendant. Wound care is also covered, and Medicare has an excellent hospice benefit (see Chapter 19).

Medicare home health services are not suited to a younger, nondisabled person who needs a few months of IV antibiotics, for example, or maybe some heparin for a blood clot. For one thing, such an individual is unlikely to be a Medicare beneficiary; for another, Medicare will not pay for medications used at home, a *big* limiting factor.

7

People with *Medicare managed care* are also eligible for home health care, though the number of home health-care agencies to choose from is more limited than that available through regular fee-for-service Medicare. Benefits and services, however, are required by law to be identical. If you are not sure whether you might have Medicare managed care, call the Social Security Administration at 1-800-772-1213. *Medicare and Home Health Care,* a publication available for free at www.medicare.gov/publications/pubs/pdf/hh.pdf, has all the information you need about Medicare home health care. General information about Medicare is available at cms.hhs.gov, or call 1-800-MEDICARE.

Medicaid

The services provided by Medicaid vary from state to state. In New York, Medicaid benefits pay for the spectrum of home health-care services, including medications and infusion: the whole gamut. When I randomly chose the Alabama Medicaid program to see what was available in states other than my own, I discovered that it, too, covered a variety of services, including home health care. Financial eligibility criteria for Medicaid, however, are strict across the board. To see what kind of services are available through Medicaid in your state, visit the U.S. Food and Drug Administration website at www.fda.gov, use the A–Z Index to find the State Department of Health Web Sites option for a direct link to all 50 state departments of health.

Private Insurance

Your health insurance might or might not cover home health care. To find out, call or visit its website (just type the company's name in your Internet search engine). Given the savings that result from shortening your hospital stay—or avoiding the hospital altogether—most insurance companies are eager to participate.

Choosing a Home Health Agency

There are many home health-care agencies across the country. Criteria to look for in choosing an agency include state licensure, accreditation by nationally recognized oversight agencies such as the Joint Committee Accrediting Health Care Organizations (JCAHO), and Medicare/Medicaid certification. Visit the National Association for Home Care at www.nahc.org for information about home care and home care agencies, including a brochure entitled *How to Choose a Home Care Provider: A Consumer's Guide,* and an easy to use agency locator with detailed information about 22,500 home care and hospice agencies. The Visiting Nurse Associations of America, at www.vnaa.org, lists over 400 visiting nurse services in 40 states.

The Mother of All Health Websites

Healthfinder, at www.healthfinder.gov, has a massive number of links to heath related websites. If you are looking for information about a specific disease, treatment, organization, health-related topic, or home care agency, Healthfinder will direct you to the right website.

Let's say you were in a car accident. You broke your leg, and now you have an infection in the bone in your thigh (*osteomyelitis*) that will take six weeks of "big gun" antibiotics to cure. You can get them in the hospital, with a roommate who snores (loudly), a flimsy cotton gown unfit to be worn in public, and the finest cuisine the hospital has to offer—or you can get them at home. You will still need to spend at least *some* time in the hospital for initial work-up and treatment, but health care at home will allow you to go home much earlier than in the past.

And if you have a heart attack, stroke, or emergency surgery that requires not only skilled nursing care, but also a doctor in the room, on the spot, and available at a moment's notice? Read on.

The following is a list of good questions and suggestions for your doctor concerning *home care:*

+ Do I have to be admitted to the hospital, or can my condition be managed at home with home care? I would like to be managed at home if at all possible.
+ If I do need to be in the hospital, would you please make sure that I am discharged to home care as soon as possible?
+ What kind of home care services do I need? What supplies will I need at home? Will I have a home attendant?
+ Will my insurance pay for home care? Will it pay for my supplies?

Chapter 2

When All Else Fails: Getting Admitted

Try as you might, there's still a good chance that a hospital stay lies in your future. If this book can't keep you out of the hospital, then it will strive to make the experience as short, painless, and safe as possible. This chapter will explore the first step, admission, and demonstrate how to get started on the right foot. But first, to better understand the process, let's look at the different kinds of hospitals in America.

Hospitals in America

Hospitals in the United States can be divided into four broad categories: general medical and surgical, specialty, psychiatric, and rehabilitation and chronic disease. They are further subdivided into for-profit and nonprofit, teaching and nonteaching, and community-based and tertiary, which are described as follows:

♦ **For-profit hospitals** are usually owned by corporations. These corporations might own several hospitals, sell stock, and issue dividends. For-profit hospitals maximize income by reducing overhead and increasing productivity, (much as other industries) to enhance their profits. Less commonly, for-profit hospitals are owned by individuals such as the doctors who practice in them.

- **Nonprofit hospitals** are owned by a nonprofit corporation, church, or the city, state, or federal government. Nonprofit hospitals do not issue stock or dividends, and any money made by providing patient care is reinvested in the institution or community (for example, by building a community health center).

For-Profit or Not-for-Profit

HCA is the largest for-profit health care company in the United States, with 200 hospitals across America, England, and Switzerland (see www.hcahealthcare.com for a list). To see if your hospital is for-profit, visit their website; a not-for-profit hospital declares this information right on its home page.

- **Teaching hospitals** are affiliated with medical, osteopathic, and nursing schools, and other health-related academic institutions such as schools for physician assistants, respiratory therapists, and so on. In addition to providing patient care, teaching hospitals train students in their chosen health care field.
- **Nonteaching hospitals** are not affiliated with academic institutions. They are usually staffed by nurses under the supervision of doctors in the community.
- **Community-based hospitals** provide general medical and surgical services to local communities.
- **Tertiary hospitals** provide specialized services for more complicated illnesses and have advanced units such as coronary and intensive care units (CCUs and ICUs), trauma units, and neonatal intensive care units (NICUs).

Note that these hospital categories are not exclusive. A community hospital can also be a teaching hospital, and a tertiary hospital—which is virtually always a teaching hospital—can provide both specialty and primary care to the people in the local community.

In addition to hospital category, the type of hospital has a big influence on the experience of patients. A large, urban, teaching facility, while similar in its fundamentals, is vastly different from a small community hospital, from the less than homey atmosphere (patients in teaching hospitals often feel they are in a fishbowl) to the types of therapies offered. Teaching hospitals, while big and impersonal, attract the best doctors and specialists, making them an indispensable source of care for the critically ill and people with complicated, rare, and esoteric conditions.

Quality of care is also influenced by an institution's type. According to the *New England Journal of Medicine*[1, 2], for-profit hospitals are not only more expensive than nonprofit facilities (in 1995, for-profit hospitals cost Medicare an additional $732 per enrollee, or $5.2 billion), but also more dangerous. The NEJM reports a 6 to 7 percent higher death rate in for-profit as compared to not-for-profit hospitals, and compared with teaching hospitals, a 25 percent higher death rate. Post-operative complications and preventable adverse events have also been found to be higher in for-profit facilities.

Your Admitting Experience

The type of hospital, then, clearly affects the kind of experience you will have during your stay. But how will it affect your *admitting* experience?

Practically speaking, your admitting experience refers to one of two things, coming into the hospital through the admitting office, which you want, or coming in through the emergency room, which you don't. Type of hospital is one influence on this process; *why* you are being admitted and *who* is admitting you are even more important. Having a doctor is the most important element of all. When you have a doctor, you are more likely to get an urgent appointment when you feel sick, to be assessed quickly, humanely, and in a private setting, and, should you require admission, you are more likely to be referred to the admitting office rather than the emergency room.

Not having a doctor, on the other hand, means going to the emergency room. Unless you are having a *true* emergency (like a heart attack or gun shot wound), this means a long and frustrating wait for a bed, little privacy, and the services of doctors and nurses who are well accustomed to the sight and sound of patients in distress. This is especially true of large, busy, urban teaching hospitals; smaller community hospitals tend to be a bit gentler.

Big Versus Small Hospitals

Once every couple of years, I work in the emergency room at Bartlett Regional Hospital in Juneau, Alaska. Bartlett, a 50-bed community hospital, is small, friendly, and provides excellent medical and surgical services. The emergency room is a dynamo, speeding patients through their x-rays and blood tests and zipping them up to a bed. In contrast to the mega-institutions in New York City, where patients in the emergency room can wait *days* for a bed, I've never seen anyone at Bartlett have to wait for more than a few hours.

Having a doctor goes a long way when wanting to avoid the ER, but it does not ensure it. For one thing, your doctor cannot be available 24 hours a day, 7 days a week; for another, an "urgent" appointment might not be soon enough. An attack of kidney stones (*nephrolithiasis*), reputed to be one of the most painful experiences a human being can suffer, merits a quick shot of morphine in the emergency room, not an urgent appointment to be seen in the office.

Another route to the emergency room, unfortunately, is being sent by your doctor as a matter of convenience. Arranging for a patient to get a bed through the admitting office requires a bit of leg work, and a full waiting room can be a strong incentive to leave the details to someone else. So if admission is the recommendation and your condition is not a true emergency, stand firm and insist you be sent to the admitting office. A quick side trip to the emergency room on your way in will be all you need to convince you that you've made the right choice.

Admitting Privileges: A Necessity

Critical to your doctor's ability to admit you to the hospital are *admitting privileges*. Admitting privileges allow him or her not only to smooth your entry through the admitting office, but also to continue to be your doctor while you are in the hospital and supervise all aspects of your care rather than entrusting you to strangers. Hospital admitting privileges are essential for the kind of soup-to-nuts health care this book advocates, and should be a make-it-or-break-it criteria when you are choosing a primary care physician.

Several other factors might also influence who takes care of you in the hospital. If you are in a critical care unit, an *intensivist* (a specialist in cardiology or pulmonology) rather than your primary care doctor will attend you. This makes sense, as the intensivist has the skills necessary for your care. Your doctor can still come to see you and advise you on treatment options, but he or she will not write orders or otherwise direct your care. When your stay is over, you might then be transferred to a non-ICU setting, where your doctor will assume control over your case.

If your doctor is affiliated with a teaching hospital, much of your care will be provided by interns and residents. An *intern* (sometimes referred to an R1) has just graduated from medical school, a *resident* (R2, R3, and so on) has completed an internship and is continuing to train in a given medical or surgical field. Collectively, interns and residents comprise the hospital's *housestaff*. Your doctor will visit at your bedside daily, and these junior physicians will be subject to his or her supervision.

Another factor critical to a smooth, quick, and painless hospital entry is bed availability. The hospital where I work, a large, nonprofit teaching hospital in the South Bronx, is often full. When it is, I have no choice but to send patients who need admission to the emergency room. Generally speaking, such bed scarcity is more common in large, urban, academic medical centers than smaller community hospitals, but this is not a hard and fast rule.

Why you are being admitted is another influence on route of entry. Conditions like pneumonia, though serious, are amenable to the calm and civility of the admitting office; you may even request a side trip home for a pair of fresh PJs and a paperback before reporting in. Heart attack and stroke, on the other hand, will land you in the ER, where your care can begin immediately, regardless of whether your doctor has admitting privileges, and regardless of bed availability. Extremely painful conditions, like kidney stones, are also appropriately referred to the ER.

Do You Need to Be Admitted?

Is this your fourth gall bladder attack? It sure is, and this one's a doozy. Darvocet, the painkiller that put you to sleep for a week after your first attack, has bounced off this one like a Ping-Pong ball off a tank. When your doctor sent you for an ultrasound at the hospital last week, the technician called his friends into the room for a look-see, whispering about "the mother of all gallstones." You dilly-dallied for as long as you could, and now it's time for an operation.

Will you tell you doctor you're ready to be admitted, or will you lay writhing on a stretcher in the emergency room for seven hours? If you've been reading this book, the former option should be yours to choose. Being in the hospital is difficult enough. Getting in should be the least of your problems. So take good care of yourself, get your screening exams, and make *sure* your doctor has admitting privileges. Your "adventure" is about to begin.

Following are some good questions and suggestions for your doctor concerning *hospital admission*:

+ What kind of hospital am I being admitted to?
+ Do you have admitting privileges at the hospital?
+ Will you be my attending doctor at the hospital? If not, who will be my attending doctor?
+ Will I be cared for by interns and residents?
+ Please make every effort to admit me through the admitting office rather than the emergency room!
+ Will I be admitted to a regular ward or to the intensive care unit? If I am in the ICU, please visit me and update me on my progress regularly!

Chapter 3

Before You Go: What Your Hospital Administrator Prefers You Don't Know

To this point, your hospital experience has been a painless one. Your doctor squeezed you into an already tight schedule to see you in his or her office, made a quick diagnosis, and referred you to your local hospital's admitting office. The admitting clerk filled out your paperwork and an orderly wheeled you up to a bed. Your nurse filled you in on the routines of the ward, a technician drew your blood and popped an IV into your arm, and you are already on a first-name basis with your roommate.

So far, so good. By all appearances, the process of being admitted to the hospital has been straightforward. Yet many forces have already come into play in your hospital stay: these powerful regulatory, legal, and financial undercurrents control much of the way contemporary hospitals function. Unfortunately, not all of these influences will be in your best interest. In keeping with the dictate that knowledge empowers self advocacy, this chapter will examine these influences to help you assure that what does happen to you in the hospital will be in your best interest.

Undercurrents in Modern Medicine: Medical Errors

The first, and most important, issue influencing your hospital stay is that of medical errors. According to *To Err Is Human,* a report by the Institute of Medicine (IOM)[1], almost 100,000 patients die in American hospitals every year as a result of the mistakes of doctors, nurses, and other hospital staff. One hundred *thousand* deaths annually—*preventable* deaths—all as a result of error. Can this be true? And if it is true, shouldn't you be running from the hospital?

The IOM's report splashed across front pages from Florida to Alaska, causing justifiable alarm among the hospital-going public. According to *CNN Headline News,* the annual number of error-induced deaths was actually 180,000. *The New York Times* compared the figure to "three fully loaded jumbo jets crashing every other day"[2], and *The Washington Post* claimed "medical errors may be the fifth leading cause of death" in America[3].

What kinds of errors did the report cite? Medical errors go far beyond surgeons forgetting to remove a pair of hemostats during surgery or doctors making the wrong diagnosis. Sloppy practice occurs, but errors happen for all kinds of reasons. A prescription is written illegibly and the wrong medication is administered. A vial of blood is mislabeled and test results are ascribed to the wrong patient. Or as medical knowledge increases, the information necessary for patient care becomes unmanageable. Medication prescribing errors are reduced when complex regimens are ordered by computer, as is the potential for dangerous interactions, but getting the necessary software up and running and integrating out-dated and incompatible data bases from different hospital departments is expensive and time consuming. And even patients themselves can cause problems. Doctors rely heavily on the information patients provide about their symptoms and medical histories. Information that is inaccurate or omitted—such as a history of drug or alcohol abuse—can easily lead to the wrong diagnosis and treatment.

The medical community was no less taken aback by the IOM's figures than the public, and follow-up studies were convened to re-examine the issue. One study, published in the *Journal of the American Medical Association (JAMA)*[4], showed clearly that the alarming figures cited by the media did not give an accurate picture of the average risk faced by the average American hospital patient—someone going into the hospital, say, for a gallbladder operation. A hundred thousand people were *not* being killed every year by medical errors. Unfortunately for the medical biz, the damage was done. The industry was put on notice, and medical error remains a prominent concern for the American public.

How have doctors and hospitals responded to this concern? Regardless of its accuracy, the IOM report was a call to action, and prevention of error has become a priority in modern medical practice. Professional organizations nationwide are moving voluntarily to confront and reduce error, and the industry's one-time tendency to protect its own by sweeping the issue under the rug has been replaced by new and increasing openness. The Agency for Healthcare Research and Quality has more information in this area at its Medical Errors and Patient Safety web page at www.ahrq.gov.

Voluntary activity is all well and good. For those who need a little more incentive, the National Conference of State Legislatures reports that 15 states now *require* that hospitals report adverse events to their state departments of health; another five and the District of Columbia have voluntary reporting systems. Part and parcel of these reporting systems is the requirement that the hospital describe actions taken to prevent similar errors in the future.

The Department of Veterans Affairs, which operates 163 hospitals and 135 nursing homes across the country, is also in on patient safety. A study by the VA's National Center For Patient Safety, for example, concluded that bar code labeling of drugs in hospitals can prevent more than 7,000 deaths a year. This system, which exemplifies the ways in which information technology can promote patient safety, uses computers to scan bar codes on patients' ID bracelets and medicine labels, and displays a warning if there is a prescribing error.

The Joint Commission on Accreditation of Healthcare Organizations (JCAHO) is the major player in hospital accreditation. Failure to win JCAHO accreditation, which is renewed every three years, will literally shut a hospital's doors (see Chapter 17 for information on how to determine if your hospital is JCAHO accredited). JCAHO takes patient safety very seriously and has established a set of "National Patient Safety Goals" certain to come up in every hospital survey. These goals range from a requirement that each patient carry at least two identifiers (for example, name and medical record number) before being given care, to marking people before surgery with labels such as "operate here" and "don't operate here" to prevent mistakes in the operating room.

Therapeutic Complications

Several years ago, a patient at a hospital in New York City died from internal bleeding after a central intravenous catheter was placed in her jugular vein. An autopsy revealed that the catheter had been placed correctly, and the death was designated by the Medical Examiner as a "therapeutic complication." This "adverse event" was reported to the state, a prolonged investigation ensued, and criteria for catheter placement were made *much* stricter. The number of catheters placed dropped dramatically, and, to date, no more patients in the hospital have died from this "therapeutic complication."

How can you prevent medical error? Participate in your care and become a full-fledged member of your error hunting team. Ask your doctors what they think is wrong with you, what kinds of diagnostic testing they are planning, what medications they have prescribed, what side effects you should watch out for, and whether those medications are safely used in combination. If your hospital does not have a computerized ordering system, ask your doctors to make sure your orders are written *legibly*, and check to assure that the medications and doses your nurse gives you are what the doctor intended. Also, make sure there is a good reason for every invasive procedure you undergo, and that goes *double* for the large bore *central lines* placed in the deep veins of your neck, upper chest, or thigh (see Chapter 1).

Don't *ever* let a doctor place a central line as a matter of convenience or because you have "difficult" veins. Most intravenous therapy does not merit a central line; let the doctors poke you with a regular IV a dozen times before even raising the subject of a central line. Chapter 17 provides more details on errors made in hospitals and how to protect yourself from them, and Chapter 21 explains how you can effectively complain if you think an error has been made during your stay.

Managed Care

Another big influence on your hospital stay is managed care. What *is* managed care? The idea, at least, is a good one. National health-care spending rose 909 percent between 1960 and 2000, from $120 billion to $1.214 trillion—almost 15 percent of the total value of goods and services produced by the country. Managed care has attempted to rein in this upward spiral, shifting payment for medical care from the time-honored method of reimbursing doctors and hospitals for services rendered—right down to the last aspirin tablet and blood test—to a system emphasizing efficiency and cost containment. Although different managed care programs vary in their specifics, most take a "case management" approach to providing service, reviewing each request before authorizing payment. Others pay a flat fee to doctors and hospitals to provide care, regardless of the actual cost of care for any individual patient.

Today, managed care is the norm. In 2001, 176.4 million Americans were enrolled in some form of managed care plan[5]. Whether this form of health insurance effectively controls costs, however, is a subject of debate. After a period of stabilization in the mid-1990s that coincided with the onset of managed care, health-care costs have resumed their rapid upward climb, especially for hospital care and prescription drugs. Advancement in high-tech, high-cost medical care is a major reason for this resurgence, along with a public and professional backlash that has led to a retreat from tightly managed care. Many people, however, also argue that the insurance industry itself is increasing costs, diverting dollars intended for health care into profits while forcing doctors and hospitals to provide more service with less money. Members of the managed care industry disagree with this viewpoint, citing narrow profit margins and maintaining that quality can be preserved and costs contained by eliminating redundancy, increasing productivity, and assuring that care meets the all-important benchmark of "medical necessity."

Got pneumonia and your doctor wants to admit you to the hospital? Your managed care company is going to be on the phone faster than you can say "penicillin." Do you *really* need to be in the hospital? Couldn't you get intravenous antibiotics at home? And what about pills? Wouldn't they do the job? In other words, is your doctor's plan for your care *medically necessary?*

I find myself on the phone three or four times a week explaining myself to a managed care nurse or doctor. Yes, my patient does need intravenous antibiotics. No, they're not well enough to go home. Yes, I'll discharge them as soon as I can, as soon as it's no longer medically necessary to keep them in the hospital. Outpatients, too, must meet the medical necessity imperative. Arranging a consultation or diagnostic procedure for a patient at one time meant picking up the phone and making an appointment. Now, a form requesting the desired service must be filled out and approval awaited as someone who has never actually laid eyes on the patient considers its merits.

To be fair, the doctors and nurses whose job it is to deal with irate physicians like me are people, too. And 9.5 times out of 10, they agree with my treatment plan and pay the hospital for its services. The hospital even has an entire department devoted to the problem, a virtual army of nurses and clerical staff who call the managed care companies to make sure the check is in the mail. And I can't think of a single test I've requested on an outpatient they wouldn't let me get. The problem is that an entire bureaucracy has been created (with money that could be spent caring for people) to play this cat-and-mouse game.

What happens to the money that the managed care companies otherwise would have spent on health care? Right into their own pockets and those of their investors. According to the *American Medical News*, stocks of 8 of the largest managed care companies were up a collective 19 percent between January and August 2002, a period in which the Dow Jones Industrial Average was down by 12 percent and the Nasdaq by 31 percent[6]. And you can bet that Wall Street does not put its faith—or its money—in an industry that is expected to be a money loser.

How Will Managed Care Influence Your Hospital Stay?

For one thing, your doctors will be under pressure to make your stay as short as possible. The less time you spend in a bed, using up medical resources and the services of doctors, nurses, and clerks, the more money the hospital will get to keep when your insurance company finally coughs up payment. Length-of-stay (LOS) is the modern day hospital administrator's mantra, and there have been dramatic reductions over the last decade. Your doctors will also have to assure that your admission is— you guessed it—medically necessary. If you're getting active treatment—medications given intravenously five or six times a day are a good example—your insurance company won't raise a fuss. If your doctor puts you in for diagnostic testing, but you're not getting *treated* for anything, that's a big managed care no-no.

To be truthful, I've never seen a patient discharged solely because of the objections of a managed care insurance company. Usually, the opposite is true; people are kept in the hospital despite the objections of managed care. Still, you might find your-self being discharged from the hospital before you feel well enough to go, or before your care is complete, and managed care might well be the reason. If this happens, talk to your doctor. You cannot be forced to leave the hospital. Tell your doctor you are concerned that you might be too sick to go home, and make sure if you do go home that you understand what medications you need to take and what signs of trouble to look out for. Get your doctor's phone number in case you have a problem, and ensure that you have an appointment for follow-up within a reasonable amount of time after discharge. Ask about having the visiting nurse service check in on you, and any home health-care services you need should be arranged well in advance of your discharge. If further diagnostic testing is planned, like a CAT scan or colonoscopy, get it scheduled *before* leaving the hospital.

If you are still dissatisfied about your planned discharge, speak to the hospital's office of patient relations or bring your complaint directly to your state department of health or JCAHO, the Joint Committee Accrediting Healthcare Organizations (see Chapter 20 for more information on how to contact JCAHO). Once again, you cannot be forced to leave the hospital; patient relations, JCAHO, or the state health department will assist you in submitting a complaint to an outside agency that has the authority to formally rescind the order for your discharge.

Getting outpatient care can also be problematic. Should you suspect that your insurance company is not cooperating in authorizing care recommended by your doctor, bone up on your medical condition, explain it to the client services representative, and *insist* you be provided the service. When this doesn't work, tell them in no uncertain terms that you *will* complain. The following are places to sound off about insurance companies that are sure to get them to sit up and listen:

- ◆ **www.state.me.us/pfr/ins/naicbro.htm.** The Maine Department of Professional and Finance Regulation, Bureau of Insurance has a very nice web page, Resolving Health Care Insurance Disputes, with a step-by-step guide on how to choose insurance, file a claim, and grieve a denial.
- ◆ **www.naic.org.** The National Association of Insurance Commissioners is a soup-to-nuts resource on health insurance, legislation, and individual insurance companies. It contains direct links to the complaint department of all 50 state insurance departments, where a complaint can be filed in a matter of minutes.

To find your specific online state insurance department, type [*your state name here*] State Insurance Department (for example, "Utah State Insurance Department") into your Internet search engine. Click the appropriate site, and you're on your way to filing an official complaint.

The Health-Care Budget Squeeze

The vagaries of managed care are only one aspect of increasing health-care costs. Health-care premiums, after rising only modestly in the 1990s, rose by 11 percent in 2001 and 13 percent in 2002, driven in part by newly resurgent health related expenditures. Employers are passing these costs to employees, raising insurance co-payments and deductibles by 30 percent over the same period. Comprehensive health insurance with no out-of-pocket expenses was once a standard benefit for just about every gainfully employed American, but no more. Co-pays for prescriptions, visits to the doctor's office, and trips to the emergency are now standard in virtually every policy.

Medicaid—which provides health coverage for more than 40 million low-income Americans, including 40 percent of births and 50 percent of nursing home care—is also under strain. Squeezed by declining tax revenues, states—which fund Medicaid jointly with the federal government—have scrambled to reduce costs by capping enrollment, raising co-pays, requiring the use of generic drugs, freezing payments to doctors and hospitals, and reducing or omitting benefits such as dental care. The Feds, facing their own budget woes, have rejected appeals for more money, instead providing wavers to the states to allow them to reduce benefits[7].

Medicare cutbacks will likewise affect more than 34 million elderly, disabled, and retired beneficiaries. Some $2.88 billion in Medicare cuts was proposed in the 2003 national budget. Payments to physicians are slated to decline by 28.1 percent between 2002 and 2005[8, 9], resulting in reimbursement levels lower than those in 1993[10]. A 15 percent cut to home health agencies is also in the works, as well as reduced funding for the training of interns and residents. The 15 percent cut scheduled (as of this writing) for October 1, 2002, would reduce funds to teaching hospitals by almost $800 million in 2003, and $4.2 billion over 5 years.

The implications of these cutbacks and retrenchment are clear. Whether you are in the hospital or the office, young or old, sick or well, care will be scarcer and more expensive, and you will be asked to shoulder an increasing percentage of the cost. Hospitals and doctors will be less willing to take on the care of the uninsured and underinsured, and, confronted by declining payments from insurance companies, Medicaid, and Medicare, they will be sending *you* the bills.

The Uninsured

Having insurance, of course, no matter how flawed, is far better than having no insurance at all. Forty-one million Americans are presently without health insurance. What happens when these people need medical care? They are admitted to the hospital later in the course of illness, their hospitalizations are longer, more complicated, more expensive, and more likely to end in death. Care is not as thorough as it is for the insured, and outpatient follow-up, including preventive care and health maintenance, is almost nonexistent. *Care Without Coverage,* a report published by the Institute of Medicine in May 2002, reviews the consequences of being uninsured in detail (visit the IOM website at www.iom.edu for a free, downloadable summary).

Medical Malpractice

As if spiraling costs, managed care, and lack of coverage wasn't enough, there's another woe facing doctors and hospitals: *malpractice.*

Medical malpractice—or "med-mal," as lawyers call it— is a $3.75 billion annual industry. According to the National Practitioner Data Bank some 149,192 malpractice payments were awarded between 1990 and the end of 2000, or roughly 15,000 per year. Because not all lawsuits are successful, the total *number* of suits over this period was quite a bit higher. The average payment for successful suits, including those settled out of court, was just shy of $249,000 in 2000. Jury awards, which run much higher than those settled out of court, increased 70 percent between 1995 and 2000, to an average of $3.5 million, with some awards running to more than $40 million[11].

How might malpractice affect your hospitalization? One possible way is by reducing the services available to you from premium saddled practitioners. Malpractice insurance rates have soared in the last decade; obstetricians in Miami and Fort Lauderdale, for example, pay $200,000 a year for coverage. Many doctors have responded by refusing to provide high-risk care, a trend that is spreading nationwide. Malpractice insurance rates for institutions have also risen; according to an American Hospital Association (AHA) survey, some 1,300 health-care institutions have made cutbacks in service directly as a result of increasing premiums and the risk of lawsuits[12].

Such reduced services can be *very* bad for your health. Time is of the essence in medical and surgical emergencies, and these service cutbacks can literally mean the difference between life and death.

High Risk = High Premiums

"High risk" medical specialties include obstetrics, orthopedics, and neurosurgery, areas in which errors can lead to dramatic, crippling injuries (e.g., lifelong problems related to a substandard delivery) and correspondingly huge malpractice awards.

Malpractice might also affect your care by causing your doctor to practice *defensive medicine*. Fearful of litigation, he or she might feel obligated to run diagnostic tests for every last problem you might suffer, no matter how unlikely they might be. This practice is a common one, replacing good judgment and effective doctor patient communication with a shotgun approach to medical care.

To avoid having your doctor practice defensive medicine, learn about your condition and communicate about your care. A trusting relationship will make you more confident that your doctor is acting in your interest, and he or she will be less worried about being sued by a suspicious and mistrustful patient. Ask whether planned testing is *really* necessary. If it isn't, a period of watchful waiting might be reasonable before scheduling complicated, expensive, and potentially harmful diagnostic procedures. Your interest should be in obtaining appropriate and thorough care, not in being run through test after test so your doctor can make sure you won't file a lawsuit.

A Critical Shortage of Nurses

Perhaps most important of all to the quality of your hospital stay is the nursing shortage. More than 126,000 nursing positions are currently unfilled in American health-care institutions, fully 75 percent of all hospital vacancies, and this number is expected to increase dramatically as aging baby boomers reach retirement age. By 2020, the United States will experience a 20 percent shortage of nurses, or some 400,000 RNs nationwide. According to JCAHO, this shortage is "a major factor in emergency department overcrowding, cancellation of elective surgeries, discontinuation of clinical services, and the limited ability of the health system to respond to any mass casualty incident. In addition, 90 percent of nursing homes report an insufficient number of nurses to provide even the most basic of care, and some home health agencies are being forced to refuse new admissions." Of some 1,600 accidental deaths and injuries that were reported by hospitals to JCAHO between January 1996 and March 2002, nursing staffing levels were a factor in 24 percent[13, 14].

What does this mean for your care? Instead of having time to spend at your bedside teaching you about your illness, your nurse will be pressured to give you your medications and move on to the next patient. You will be spending considerably less time with one of the best sources of information and care the hospital has to offer, and many of the most important elements of your stay, such as administering meds and putting in IVs, will be performed by lesser trained hospital staff such as *licensed practice nurses* (LPN) and *patient care technicians* (PCT) (see Chapter 7). You might have difficulty getting your medication on time and your pain medications might arrive an hour or more late.

Pain, Pain, Go Away

Waiting for pain medicine is one of the biggest complaints of hospital patients. If you have a painful condition (or if you expect to have pain, for example, after surgery), ask your doctor to arrange for *patient controlled analgesia* (see Chapter 14) so you don't have to wait for a nurse to get relief.

A Mountain of Paperwork

Increased governmental oversight, the growth of managed care, and gains in the malpractice industry might—in the opinion of some—have improved patient safety and increased efficiency in the delivery of medical care, but they have also created an avalanche of paperwork. In a report commissioned by the American Hospital Association[15], it was estimated that paperwork adds at least 30 minutes to every hour of hands on care provided for the average patient, and, in some settings, an *hour* to every hour of care. The rules and instructions for Medicare and Medicaid alone run some 130,000 pages—three times the size of the tax code. In addition, some 30 federal health-care regulatory agencies have their own paperwork requirements, as do state and local agencies and accreditation authorities. Lawyers, who scrutinize every last detail of a patient's records during a lawsuit, add another paperwork pressure.

You're *in* ... Now What?

You've only just gotten a room, and there are already a dozen "hidden" issues to bear in mind. If your doctor doesn't know the answers to the questions at the end of this chapter, ask for the *administrator-on-duty* or *patient representative* to provide the information you need.

A hospital that is strapped for money, cutting back on services, subject to regulatory oversight from state or voluntary agencies, or scrambling for nursing coverage might be one you want to avoid (although there's nothing like a state investigation to make an institution more attentive to its patients than ever). At the absolute minimum, insist that your doctor keep you informed about all aspects of your care: the diagnoses being considered, the work-up and therapy being planned, the care you will need after discharge, and the *risks* that are a part of your care.

Following are some good questions and suggestions for your doctor concerning *hidden influences in your hospital stay:*

♦ Will my medication orders be written by hand or computer? Please make sure if they are written by hand that they are legible!

♦ Please check for dangerous interactions between my medications.

♦ Have there been any serious errors or preventable patient deaths recently in this hospital? How did the hospital respond to these events?

♦ What kinds of quality improvement activities have recently been conducted in this hospital?

♦ Has there been a recent JCAHO survey? How did the hospital do? In what areas was it cited?

♦ Has my admission been approved by my insurance company?

♦ Has the hospital recently eliminated any services I might need?

♦ Does the hospital have a nursing shortage? How many patients are on my ward, and how many nurses care for them?

♦ If I have serious pain, please provide me with *patient controlled analgesia* so I do not have to wait for a nurse to get relief.

Chapter 4

Nine Hours on a Molded Orange Plastic Chair: The Emergency Room

Part 1 of this book introduced you to ways of staying out of the hospital. For those who *must* be admitted, Chapter 2 reviewed referral through the admitting office, and Chapter 3 some of the hidden influences on modern hospital function. If you have to be admitted, you have now arrived in a bed after a calm and civilized appointment with your doctor, a quick visit to the admitting office, and a wheelchair ride upstairs with an orderly. Shortly, your doctor will come to your room to interview and examine you, explain what is wrong and what should be done, and begin your diagnostic work-up and therapy.

The real world might not be so gentle. It's possible that you don't have a doctor, that you were unable to get an appointment, or that your medical condition was too urgent to wait. Maybe you developed sudden, severe pain and called an ambulance. Worse, you suffered chest pain, a stroke, or any of dozens of other medical or surgical emergencies that merit an immediate call to 911.

Whatever the cause, you wound up in the emergency room. This chapter examines the emergency room experience in depth, in the hope of helping you avoid the ER if at all possible, and to help you get through the ordeal if there is no way to avoid it.

The Emergency Room: Hollywood Versus Reality

Dramatized by countless television shows and movies, the emergency room is fixed in the public consciousness; chaotic, noisy, and filled with wounded humanity. Harsh florescent lights illuminate ceaseless action, accompanied by a tumble of voices, cries, and the hum of machinery. Gunshot victims are rushed down hallways by haggard doctors and nurses, and heart attack patients are shocked to life in tense, emotional scenes.

The reality of the emergency room is much more mundane. Many emergency rooms, especially those in large, urban, academic medical centers, function largely as clinics, grinding out care for the poor and uninsured, patching up the chronically ill, triaging the sick for admission, and referring the not-so-sick for care at a later date. There are heart attack and trauma victims, too, and dramatic, life-and-death scenarios, but this is more the exception than the rule. The emergency room is the scene of steady action and small victories—cuts repaired, fractures cast, infections treated—more often than sudden, life-changing events.

For many, especially those without insurance, the emergency room is a major source of medical care. A 1998 study conducted in New York City[1] showed that nearly 75 percent of people visiting the emergency room had nonurgent conditions or urgent conditions that could have been treated in a doctor's office. Another 7 percent had conditions that needed ER care but that were preventable, such as asthma flare-ups or diabetes. People who relied on the ER as their sole source of care lacked the continuity that is so important to health maintenance and disease management, and many ultimately got sicker and used much more expensive and time-consuming services.

Another study (partly conducted at the Bronx, New York, hospital where I work) examined the problem of inappropriate ER utilization in more depth. Not surprisingly, it found that one of the most important reasons people sought ER care for less-than-urgent conditions was lack of insurance. Uninsured people were 3 times as likely as those with Medicaid (15 versus

5 percent) to cite health-care access problems as their reason for going to the emergency room, and fully half reported that they did not have a regular doctor or clinic[2].

What does this mean for you? Health maintenance and disease management in collaboration with a primary care doctor is one of the most important means of avoiding the emergency room. Whether you are well or facing a chronic illness, having a doctor is the best means of staying at home.

But let's face it. Whether you have a doctor or not, a trip to the emergency room is probably in your future.

A Visit to the Emergency Room

To be prepared for that day, when you wonder whether you should go to the emergency room, here is a list of good and not-so-good reasons to go.

Good reasons to go to the emergency room include ...

+ Loss of consciousness.
+ Signs of heart attack such as pressure, fullness, squeezing, or pain in chest, and chest pain associated with lightheadedness or pounding of the heart (palpitations).
+ Signs of a stroke, including sudden weakness or numbness of the face or one side of the body, sudden loss of vision or speech, trouble talking or understanding words, new and severe headaches, severe dizziness, unsteadiness of balance, and unexpected falls.
+ Shortness of breath.
+ Bleeding that does not stop after 10 minutes of direct pressure.
+ Severe pain.
+ Poisoning or overdose. Call your local poison control center for potentially lifesaving advice on treatment at home. Keep a bottle of Syrup of Ipecac in your medicine cabinet in case they advise you to induce vomiting, and activated charcoal for leeching poisons from your blood and intestines.

+ An allergic reaction to an insect bit or sting, or to a medication, especially if breathing is difficult.
+ A major injury.
+ Unexplained stupor or disorientation.
+ Coughing up, vomiting, or passing blood in the stool.
+ Persistent vomiting.
+ Suicidal or homicidal feelings.
+ High fever, especially in a child under age three, the elderly, or people who are immunocompromised (e.g., those with AIDS, those on cancer chemotherapy, and those who have had organ transplants).

Not so good reasons to go to the emergency room include ...

+ Earache.
+ Minor cuts.
+ Minor animal bites (see your physician—a rabies or tetanus shot might be needed).
+ Sunburn or minor burns.
+ A minor skin rash.
+ Sexually transmitted diseases.
+ Colds and cough, sore throat, flu.

Now, let's take the following common scenario as an example of *your* ER visit and follow it from beginning to end.

For a day or two, you've had a vague discomfort in your stomach. Today, the pain got much worse, and you vomited the few spoonfuls of soup you tried to eat for lunch. When you took your temperature this afternoon, it was 100.5. You called your doctor and he advised you to stay home, drink clear fluids, and take Tylenol for pain and fever. If the pain got much worse, though, or if you had a high temperature, he told you to go to the emergency room.

Your spouse drove you to the ER at the nearby academic medical center when your temp hit 104, leaving a message with your doctor's answering service that you were going.

What's the diagnosis?

You *might* have appendicitis.

What's next?

We will return to your dilemma shortly. But first, let's go over a few ER basics.

ER Basics #1: Triage

As soon as you arrive in the emergency room, whether it is by ambulance, cab, or walking in off the street, you will be seen by a nurse and *triaged*. The nurse will record your complaint, take your blood pressure, pulse, respiratory rate, and temperature (*vital signs*), and assess the urgency of your condition. If your problem is life threatening, like a heart attack, you will be immediately seen by a doctor. If your condition is not life threatening but still serious and painful, like an attack of kidney stones, you will be prioritized for urgent attention, but—depending on how busy things are—you might not be seen as quickly as you would be were your condition more serious. If your problem is less urgent yet, but still very real and discomforting—like a high fever and a bad cough—you are further down the list. Other conditions will merit you an even lower space, and you might wait so long that you eventually give up and go home. The pain you started having after you threw out your back two years ago, for example, is *not* an emergency—even if it's getting worse, and even if you haven't slept in a week because of it. And six hours on the molded orange plastic chair in the emergency room waiting area is not what you need to start feeling better.

ER Basics #2: Vital Signs

Among the most important factors in determining how sick you are your *vital signs* (see the previous paragraph). Very low blood pressure—*shock*, characterized by weakness, pallor (paleness), sweaty skin, and a rapid heart rate—is an ominous sign of unstable and dangerous conditions such as blood loss (external and internal), sepsis (blood infection), and heart failure.

Rapid heart rate (*tachycardia,* in excess of 100 beats per minute) might also be seen in cardiac arrhythmias (which might be rapid *or* slow), as well as less worrisome conditions such as fever and anxiety. Regardless, it is an alarming sign that merits urgent attention. A rapid respiratory rate (greater than 20) is also a worrisome sign, as is a high fever.

Triage involves more than just taking your vital signs. Why you have come to the ER is another factor. This information, called your "chief complaint," or, more simply, your "complaint," also helps determine how sick you are. This chapter will review some of the more common "chief complaints" and how they are likely to be triaged. Although these guidelines are not exhaustive—*anyone* who believes he or she might be suffering from a medical emergency should immediately call 911 or report to the nearest emergency room—they might help you understand how long you will have to wait for a given complaint, and whether you are likely to be admitted to the hospital.

ER Basics #3: Common Conditions

The following are common, day-to-day symptoms and medical problems that bring thousands of Americans to the emergency room every day.

Chest Pain

Chest pain is *always* taken seriously in the emergency room because of the possibility that it represents a heart attack. Cardiac chest pain is typically dull, achy, or squeezing, located in the midchest, and associated with shortness of breath. It can extend into the neck, jaw, shoulders, or arms, and might be accompanied by a feeling of numbness, especially in the left arm. There might also be nausea, sweating, and pallor (paleness). Often, cardiac chest pain is made worse by exertion (such as climbing stairs), and better by resting. *Atypical chest pain* is that which differs from this pattern, but which also an represent a heart attack (for example, pain that is burning or feels like indigestion rather than pressure, is located in the upper abdomen rather than the chest, or occurs at rest rather than with exertion). Chest pain is more likely to be a sign of a heart attack in people with cardiac risk factors such as a family history of heart disease, obesity, high blood pressure, diabetes, cigarette smoking, and high blood cholesterol, and in those who are middle aged. People who are younger and without risks for heart disease and who have chest pain made worse by coughing or taking a deep breath might have *costochondritis:* inflammation of the ribs, cartilage, or muscles of the rib cage, a common cause of noncardiac chest pain.

Chest pain will be triaged for immediate attention by the triage nurse, who will record a tracing of the electrical activity of the heart (*electrocardiogram,* or *EKG*) and show it to a doctor. The doctor will assess the EKG for signs of heart attack, and, taken together with a brief description of the chest pain and the patient's underlying risk for heart disease, decide on the urgency of further evaluation.

Shortness of Breath

Shortness of breath is also a very serious symptom. Shortness of breath can result from heart attack, congestive heart failure, asthma, chronic bronchitis, emphysema, pulmonary embolism (a blood clot in the lungs), pneumonia, and many other conditions.

People who are having an asthma attack are ushered immediately into the emergency room to an area reserved for the treatment of this condition (the "asthma area") and given inhaled medications to relieve the wheezing and shortness of breath that characterizes this condition.

Pain

Pain is a very common symptom in the emergency room. Pain from trauma, especially open fractures, lacerations, or active bleeding, merits rapid attention; how lesser degrees of pain are triaged depends on severity and cause.

Location of pain is an important consideration. Chest pain, as described previously, is taken very seriously. Abdominal pain also merits thorough consideration, though it will not necessarily be triaged for immediate assessment. Abdominal pain located in the upper mid-abdomen, made worse by meals, and present over a long period of time, for example, is a common condition, often caused by irritation of the stomach from excess acid (*gastritis*). Ulcers of the stomach or small intestine (*gastric and duodenal ulcers*) might also cause upper abdominal pain. Though serious and painful, these problems might lead to your spending more time in the emergency room waiting area or sweating it out on a gurney than you would like.

Pain From One to Ten

Many doctors and nurses assess the severity of pain by asking patients to rate their pain on a scale from zero to ten, with zero being no pain, and ten being "the worst pain you've ever experienced in your life." Recently, pain management experts have also begun to employ a four-level scale, "none, mild, moderate, severe," which is easier to use and just as accurate in "measuring" pain.

Abdominal pain might also be caused by ...

- *Gallstones* (*cholelithiasis*), with pain in the upper right abdomen.
- *Appendicitis*, with pain in the lower right abdomen.
- *Diverticulae* (small, baglike pouches in the wall of the large intestine, common in the elderly), with pain in the lower left abdomen.
- *Pancreatitis* (inflammation of the pancreas), with severe, burning mid-abdominal pain that might bore though to the back.
- *Kidney stones and kidney infection* (*nephrolithiasis and pyelonephritis*), with pain on either side of the mid-lower back, sometimes reaching down and around to the groin.

These are not hard and fast rules, and there are many other causes of abdominal pain. Appendicitis, for example, might cause pain in the mid-abdomen, and gallstones can cause pain in the lower abdomen. Most cases of abdominal pain will merit examination by a surgeon, but you can expect to wait a while, especially if your vital signs are stable and the ER is busy.

Relieve Your Pain

The widely held misconception that people with abdominal pain must be assessed by a surgeon before effective relief can be provided still holds sway in many emergency rooms, and the staff might skimp on pain relievers until the surgeon arrives. This practice has been proven unnecessary[3], and you are in the right in requesting relief.

Chronic pain, caused by anything from a slipped disc to *fibromyalgia,* is another frequent reason for emergency room visits. Fibromyalgia, which tends to strike women, causes fatigue, body aches, and *lancinating* (lightninglike) pain. Chronic low back pain is another common symptom. Unfortunately, these problems are not regarded as urgent, and the individual who comes to the busy emergency room seeking relief after weeks, months, or years of suffering is going to be spending time cooling his or her heels in the waiting area.

Headache

Criteria to triage headache include its severity, whether there have been similar headaches in the past, whether the headaches are associated with nausea and vomiting, blurred or double vision, and whether neurologic abnormalities such as weakness or numbness on one side of the face or body and unsteadiness of balance (that might be a sign of a stroke, bleeding, or a mass in the brain) co-exist. Patients who describe "the worst headache I've ever had in my life; completely different from anything I've had before" are rapidly triaged to be seen by a doctor.

People with migraine headache, on the other hand, especially those little different from migraines they've had in the past, are likely to spend many unhappy hours on the molded orange plastic chair in the waiting room. Migraines, throbbing, one-sided headaches that are made worse by light and noise and are often accompanied by nausea and vomiting, might be excruciatingly painful, but they are not considered emergencies.

Headache resulting from hypertension might cause throbbing pain at the base of the skull. Very elevated blood pressure will be triaged for urgent attention. Stage III hypertension, with a diastolic blood pressure in excess of 110 (and as high as 150 or more), might be accompanied by neurologic abnormalities, *altered mental status,* and swelling of the back of the eye (*retina*), which is visible with an ophthalmoscope. Untreated, malignant hypertension can lead to stroke and permanent damage to the kidneys, heart, and other organs.

Pain at the base of the skull can also be a sign of meningitis, especially when accompanied by fever. Affected patients complain of stiffness and neck pain and might have a red, speckled rash. An infection of the covering of the brain and spinal cord (*meninges*), meningitis, when bacterial, is a medical emergency that requires immediate treatment with intravenous antibiotics.

Altered Mental Status

Altered mental status (AMS) refers to a change in a person's thought patterns or level of consciousness. People with AMS might be confused, agitated, lethargic, obtunded, or comatose. *Lethargic* people are sleepy but easily aroused; *obtunded* people require constant stimulus to stay awake. AMS is common in drug and alcohol intoxication, head trauma, and a variety of medical conditions that affect the brain, including malignant hypertension, meningitis, stroke, brain tumors, and blood clots.

Epilepsy (Seizures)

Seizures are also evaluated on an emergency basis. Characterized by sudden loss of consciousness, violent twitching of the body, and loss of bladder control, a *generalized*, or *tonic-clonic* seizure is a frightening sight. Most seizures are caused by *epilepsy* (seizure disorder), a chronic illness that is controlled by taking daily medications.

Loss of Consciousness

Sudden, unexpected lethargy or loss of consciousness (*syncope*) might result from a simple (or common) faint (*vasovagal syncope*) due to emotional distress. Insulin overdose and very low blood sugar (*hypoglycemia*) is a common cause of loss of consciousness in diabetics, usually preceded by confusion, sweatiness, weakness, and palpitations (the sensation of a rapid, pounding heart rate). Severe dehydration or illness is another common cause of lethargy and loss of consciousness. A *concussion* is a brief loss of consciousness resulting from head trauma.

Fever

Like pain, fever is common in the emergency room. Fever can be a sign of a minor problem or a life threatening illness. A young, healthy individual with fever but no signs of a serious infection, for example, is likely to be sent to the waiting room before being seen by a doctor. *Febrile* people (those with fever) with chronic illnesses such as diabetes, heart disease, or kidney failure, on the other hand, are more likely to have a serious infection. Elderly people also merit closer attention. Some of the more common diagnoses considered in the emergency room include pneumonia, urinary tract infections, and meningitis, though the majority of ER patients have little more than a viral illness such as a cold or the flu.

Minor Bleeding, Burns, and Trauma

Most minor bleeding is easily managed at home by applying direct pressure to the wound with a clean gauze or washcloth for ten minutes. If this doesn't control the bleeding, or if a cut is sufficiently deep, a trip to the ER for stitches (*sutures*) might be necessary. Minor trauma and burns are likewise subject to basic first-aid treatment at home.

A sprain is an injury such as a bruise or a minor tear to a ligament (a band of tough, fibrous tissue that connects a bone to a bone). Most sprains should be x-rayed to make sure a bone isn't broken. If you have a sprain and can be seen by your doctor for an x-ray, do so. If not, go to the ER, but plan on spending the better part of the day sitting around waiting for one, and then another few hours waiting for the result.

Gastrointestinal Bleeding

Vomiting blood or digested blood—dark material that looks like coffee grounds (*coffee ground emesis*)—should prompt an *immediate* call to 911. Passing blood or purplish black material from the rectum (*bright red blood per rectum,* BRBPR, and *melena*) also merits an urgent trip to the ER. Streaks of blood noted on stool (or toilet paper) are less worrisome and are usually due to hemorrhoids.

Poisoning, Overdose, and Drug or Alcohol Intoxication

People who overdose on poisons, prescription pills, and other substances are triaged for immediate attention. Medications involved in overdoses range from over-the-counter pain relievers and cold preparations to prescription antidepressants, antibiotics, analgesics, and virtually any other medication that can be found in the medicine cabinet. Nonfood, nonmedication substances, such as Clorox and other household cleansers and solvents, are also accidentally ingested and used in suicide attempts.

Acetaminophen, the active ingredient in more than 200 OTC cold, headache, and pain relief preparations, including Tylenol, can cause deadly liver damage and is one of the most common substances involved in overdoses. Data collected by the American Association of Poison Control Centers estimates that 108,102 calls were made to Poison Control Centers in 1999 because of acetaminophen overdose, and the National Hospital Ambulatory Care Survey and National Hospital Discharge Survey report almost 57,000 acetaminophen-related annual emergency room visits, 26,000 hospitalizations, and 458 deaths.

How does acetaminophen cause so many poisonings and deaths? One reason is that acetaminophen is contained in so many pain, flu, and cold preparations that people accidentally overdose when they take more than one medication at a time. And because the toxic dose is not much higher than the therapeutic dose (5 grams in 24 hours might cause toxicity; the recommended maximum daily dose is 4 grams), accidental over-dose with a single agent is not difficult. Even people who over-dose intentionally often do not understand the drug's dangers. The Food and Drug Administration estimates that of the 57 to 74 percent of overdoses that are intentional, many are "cries for help" among people who do not know they are dealing with such a toxic and potentially fatal medication[4].

Responding to the dangers posed by acetaminophen, the FDA in September 2002 recommended bold face labeling on medica-tions containing the ingredient, warnings that taking more than the recommended dose can cause serious liver damage[5].

Ibuprofen, the main ingredient in Motrin and Advil, and *naproxyn,* found in Aleve and Naprosyn, are also common OTC analgesics. In 1998, the AAPCC reported 52,751 acute overdoses of ibuprofen, 13,519 hospitalizations, and 4 deaths. Many *more* hospitalizations and deaths are caused when the drug is taken in *recommended* doses, especially over a period of weeks or months. A significant cause of stomach ulcers, gastrointestinal bleeding, and kidney damage, ibuprofen and related drugs used in therapeutic doses caused 100,000 hospital-izations in 1998, and 10,000—yes, ten *thousand*—fatalities[6].

Iron is another common poison. The FDA reported that 110,000 children were poisoned by iron between 1986 and 1997. Of these, 35 died, making iron overdose a leading cause of poisoning deaths in children under age 6. The iron prepara-tions that lead to poisoning range from OTC multivitamin and mineral supplements for children to high-potency prescription formulations for pregnant women[7]. Children or adults who overdose on iron should be taken *immediately* to the ER.

Alcoholics are frequent emergency room users, when they are intoxicated and brought in off the street by the police and EMS, when they are injured, and when they attempt to go "cold turkey" and develop *alcohol withdrawal syndrome* (which is called delirium tremens, or DTs in its most severe form). Char-acterized by tremulousness, agitation, confusion, and auditory and visual hallucinations (pink elephants), DTs can lead to convulsions, vomiting, *aspiration* (the inhaling of stomach contents and saliva), and death. Alcoholics are attended promptly in the emergency room, if only to assure that they are stable and to let them sleep it off before being referred for detox.

Overdose with "street" drugs such as heroin and cocaine is also common. Heroin overdose can lead to respiratory depression and death; cocaine overdose might cause fatal heart attack. Marijuana is an extremely rare cause of acute toxicity.

Getting Clean and Sober

"Detox" is the process of getting an alcoholic through the 7- to 10-day period of high risk for developing alcohol withdrawal syndrome (AWS) and delirium tremens after his or her last drink. AWS is treated with sedatives such as Valium or Librium. Once complete, detox is followed by "rehab," a much longer period in which the alcoholic learns to live without drinking.

Should you suffer from an overdose or intoxication, call your local poison control center for advice *after* calling 911. To find the poison control center nearest you call 1-800-222-1222. Make sure to have some *Syrup of Ipecac* on hand in case the poison control center recommends that you induce vomiting. You should also keep some activated charcoal in the medicine cabinet. Mixed with water or soda, activated charcoal absorbs toxic substances from the blood and intestines for excretion in the stool. See the following instructions on how to use Syrup of Ipecac and activated charcoal, and do *not* use either substance without first calling your doctor or local poison control center.

How to Administer Syrup of Ipecac to Induce Vomiting

1. Call your local poison control center (1-800-222-1222) to make *sure* vomiting is recommended after an overdose. Syrup of Ipecac is available without prescription.

2. If vomiting *is* recommended, give: 15 milliliters (3 teaspoons or 1 tablespoon) and half glass or 4 ounces water for children, or 30 milliliters (6 teaspoons or 2 tablespoons) with or 8 to 12 ounces of water for adults.
3. Repeat in a half hour if vomiting (*emesis*) has not occurred.

How to Administer Activated Charcoal

1. Call your local poison control center to make sure that charcoal is recommended after an overdose. Activated charcoal is also available without prescription.
2. Give 1 gram per kilogram of body weight of activated charcoal mixed with 8 ounces water or soda to children, or roughly 25 to 50 grams for children weighing approximately 50 to 100 pounds.
3. Give 25 to 100 grams of activated charcoal mixed in 8 to 16 ounces water or soda to adolescents and adults weighing from 100 to 250 pounds.
4. Do not give charcoal within 2 hours of a dose of Ipecac.

Do not give Syrup of Ipecac or activated charcoal unless the poisoning victim is fully conscious!

Do not give Syrup of Ipecac or activated charcoal to someone who is having difficulty breathing!

Always call your doctor or local poison control center for advice before administering activated charcoal or Syrup of Ipecac!

Allergic Reactions

Allergy to insect bites, foods (especially peanuts and shellfish), and medications are common, resulting in hives, rash, swelling of the face, wheezing, and difficulty breathing. Mild allergic reactions will not merit urgent attention in the ER, but swelling of the neck and face associated with shortness of breath (*anaphylaxis*) will be urgently triaged. If you have a dangerous allergy, talk to your doctor about getting a pre-packed syringe of *epinephrine* (*Epipen*) to keep with you in case you are accidentally exposed to the allergen. Epinephrine can be a lifesaver should you develop swelling, shortness of breath, or wheezing.

People with severe allergies should also wear medical alert bracelets to warn health-care providers of their allergy should they be brought unconscious into an ER. This will help prevent their being inadvertently administered the wrong medication.

Psychiatric Illness

Psychiatric conditions seen in the ER include depression, schizophrenia, and mania. Overtly psychotic patients, who are unable to understand the consequences of their own actions and require hospitalization for their own protection, are often brought in by friends, family, or the police. Homicidal or suicidal thoughts (*ideation*) are taken very seriously by the psychiatric staff.

Keep in mind that the decision to hold someone against his or her will is a serious one. That a patient "does not understand the consequences of their own actions" is a judgment made by two doctors before a patient may be involuntarily committed to a psychiatric facility.

What to Expect at the Emergency Room

When last we checked, your spouse had dropped you off at the emergency room, leaving you with the triage nurse, and gone to park the car. The belly pain you'd been having had gotten suddenly worse, and you had a fever of 104. You put in a call to your doctor to let him know you were headed to the ER, and he promised he'd get a surgeon in to see you. Now what?

After signing in at the registration desk (where a clerk will record your address, phone number, next of kin, emergency contact information, employer, type of health insurance, and policy number), the triage nurse will record your vital signs and your chief complaint. If the hospital is a small community hospital and the emergency room is not busy, you will be ushered inside, put on a gurney, and asked to change into a gown. If the emergency room is in a large urban medical center, the wait to see a doctor might be anywhere from a few minutes to a few hours, and possibly even longer if your vital signs are stable. Waiting, unfortunately, is the name of the game in the emergency room. Unless you are *really* sick, as in having a heart attack or another immediate, life-threatening emergency, you're going to spend a good amount of time waiting for things to happen.

Your initial interview with the doctor will be succinct and to the point. You will be asked your age, whether you have any chronic illnesses or have had surgery, what medications you take, your allergies, whether you smoke, drink, or use drugs, and, if you are a woman, how many pregnancies you have had and when you had your last menstrual period. Depending on the nature of your complaint, you might be asked a variety of related questions, such as your sexual history and whether you have ever had a sexually transmitted disease, your HIV status, your living conditions, and details of previous medical tests and hospitalizations. Questions will be directed both to your chief complaint and a "review of systems" covering other areas of your body (heart, lungs, nervous system, and so on).

You will be interviewed and examined in a semi-private setting, with a curtain separating you from the person on the next stretcher. Because there is a suspicion of appendicitis, the physical exam (*PE*) will include a rectal examination. Then you will undergo testing to "work-up" your complaint. You will have an IV put in your arm, blood tests drawn, and x-rays. In your case, a CT scan will be ordered in addition to the usual chest x-ray for a closer look at your appendix (see Chapter 8 for more information on diagnostic testing).

At this early stage of your emergency room visit, your pain has been assessed by the emergency room doctor. Remember that you should not be kept waiting for the surgeon before getting relief. As mentioned, many doctors believe that pain is a necessary diagnostic sign and will allow it to go unrelieved until the surgeon has made an assessment. Once again, this is not true, and you should *insist* on relief.

If you're lucky, only two hours will have passed between reporting to the triage nurse and getting a CAT scan. If you're really lucky, and the ER is in the middle of a down time, only an hour will have gone by. But don't worry, you're well on your way. The doctor has started a diagnostic work-up, your IV is in, and the blood tests are in the laboratory. You've had a chest x-ray and a CT scan. You've made a fuss and been given pain relief, and ... here comes the surgeon.

What happens next? A bit of waiting is still in the offing. Blood tests and x-rays take a while to generate results, and the surgeon is going to want to see them before making the decision to take you to the operating room. It's possible that you will not be taken to the operating room at all, but admitted for further observation and testing. Several more hours in the ER are in your future, or, if there's a bed available, you'll be taken upstairs. But what do you care? The surgeon saw you, made a tentative diagnosis, and gave you *more* morphine. Now, you don't care *what* happens.

What happens next is that you will sign your life away, and be admitted to the hospital. Chapter 5 will show you how.

Following are some good questions and suggestions for your doctor concerning *the emergency room:*

+ Do I *have* to go the emergency room? If possible, I prefer that my condition be taken care of in your office with close follow-up by telephone and revisiting.
+ Is the emergency room likely to be busy and crowded?
+ Will I have to wait a long time to be seen by a doctor and for x-rays and blood tests?
+ What will be done for me in the emergency room?
+ Will my pain (or other discomfort) be attended promptly in the emergency room?
+ Please call ahead to notify the ER doctor of my arrival!
+ How long will I have to stay in the emergency room?
+ Will I have to wait for a bed for a long time? Please call ahead to arrange for a bed for me!

Chapter 5

Sign on the Dotted Line, Please: Informed Consent, Patient's Rights, and Other Legal Matters

One of the first things that will be asked of you in the hospital is your formal consent to be treated. A form, vaguely worded and weighted in favor of the hospital, will be shoved under your nose saying that you consent to be treated in any way the hospital deems appropriate. Given the pain you're having, or the fever, or the hacking cough, you'll probably go ahead and sign it. The goal of this form is to protect the hospital from the claim that you were treated against your will, and, to a lesser extent, to provide them some cover in case things turn out badly for you.

Practically speaking, though, such general "consent to treatment" forms afford hospitals little real protection. Legally speaking, you have not consented to *all* possible treatments, and you certainly haven't consented to malpractice. So go ahead and sign. You will still have the ability to take legal action if something awful happens (given the volume of malpractice suits, these forms don't seem to have stopped anyone so far), and, besides, your biggest concern right now is getting better, not sweating the details of your opportunity to seek redress should things go awry.

The Patient's Bill of Rights

While the "consent to treatment" form emphasizes the rights of hospitals, it is the right of *patients* that have grown the most in the last few decades. The "Patient's Bill of Rights," a document which should be given to you when you are admitted (and which also should be posted at the entrance to each of the hospital's wards), lists these rights. Central to it's premise, and a fundamental theme of this book, is your legal prerogative to receive information about your medical condition, participate in making decisions about your care, and, should you not be included in the decision making process in a way you see fit, be provided an effective means of complaining, either to the hospital itself or, if necessary, to outside authorities. It is your right, in short, to direct the course of your care in the hospital and to be given the information you need to do so.

Patient's rights are guaranteed by law in most states. Though variable in their specifics, each of these statutes focuses on the right of patients to choose their own care. (To see if your state has a bill of rights, visit your state health department's website.) The Federal government requires compliance with a similar bill of rights as a condition for participation in Medicare, making it applicable to every hospital, nursing home, institutional hospice, and home care agency in the country. What follows is the New York State bill of rights, which is representative of bills found in other states and the Federal bill establishing requirements for participation in Medicare[1].

The "Patient's Bill of Rights" for New York State

As a patient in a New York State hospital you have the right, consistent with law, to the following:

1. Understand and use these rights. If for any reason you do not understand or you need help, the hospital must provide assistance, including an interpreter.
2. Receive treatment without discrimination as to race, color, religion, sex, national origin, disability, sexual orientation, or source of payment.

3. Receive considerate and respectful care in a clean and safe environment, free of unnecessary restraints.
4. Receive emergency care if you need it.
5. Be informed of the name and position of the doctor who will be in charge of your care in the hospital.
6. Know the names, positions, and functions of any hospital staff involved in your care in the hospital and refuse their treatment, examination, or observation.
7. A no smoking room.
8. Receive complete information about your diagnosis, treatment, and prognosis.
9. Receive all the information that you need to give informed consent for any proposed procedure or treatment. This information shall include the possible risks and benefits of procedure or treatment.
10. Receive all the information that you need to give informed consent for an order not to resuscitate. You also have the right to designate an individual to give this consent for you if you are too ill to do so. If you would like additional information, please ask for a copy of the pamphlet, "Do Not Resuscitate Order—A Guide for Patients and Families".
11. Refuse treatment and be told what effect this may have on your health.
12. Refuse to take part in research. In deciding whether or not to participate, you have the right to a full explanation.
13. Privacy while in the hospital and confidentiality of all information and records regarding your care.
14. Participate in all decisions about your treatment and discharge from the hospital. The hospital must provide you with a written discharge plan and written description of how you can appeal your discharge.
15. Review your medical record without charge. Obtain a copy of your medical record for which the hospital can charge a reasonable fee. You cannot be denied a copy solely because you cannot afford to pay.
16. Receive an itemized bill and explanation of all charges.

17. Complain without fear of reprisals about the care and services you are receiving and to have the hospital respond to you and if you request it, a written response. If you are not satisfied with the hospital's response, you can complain to the New York State Health Department. The hospital must provide you with the Health Department's telephone number.

18. Authorize those family members and other adults who will be given priority to visit, consistent with your ability to receive visitors.

19. Make known your wishes in regard to anatomical gifts. You may document your wishes in your health care proxy or on a donor card, available from the hospital.

The patient's bill of rights is a serious document, intended to protect *your* right to decide what will happen to *your* body in the hospital. Use it!

Advance Directives and the Health-Care Proxy

Also included in the documents provided you at admission will be forms intended to allow you to choose the kind of care you want at the end-of-life. Referred to as *advance directives,* these documents, usually either *health-care proxy* or *living will* forms (depending on your state) are almost always used by people who wish to instruct their doctors not to engage in "heroics" should they become gravely and irreversibly ill and be unable to advocate for themselves (for example, because they are in a coma and on a respirator). Advance directives should be completed by *everyone*, regardless of whether he or she is admitted to the hospital. Care at the end-of-life-will be discussed much more in Chapter 19, along with sample advance directive forms.

Informed Consent

Most people go to the hospital for a well-defined problem, get better, and go home. Many need diagnostic and therapeutic procedures that carry some degree of risk; it is in these situations that *informed consent* is important.

What is informed consent? At one time, the process was little more than a perfunctory recitation of the risks and benefits of a given procedure, delivered by a disinterested doctor and accompanied a hurried request for a signature. "You need to have your gallbladder out, there could be a little bleeding, sign here please. And you might get an infection, too. Here's a pen."

Get Second Opinions

Consider getting a second opinion before consenting to any procedure that you are unsure about. Also make sure to ask your doctor the questions listed at the end of this chapter. Then ask yourself if you have had enough time to make a clear-headed and unpressured decision.

Today, informed consent is more of a conversation than a recitation, and the protections offered to both doctor and patient are substantial. Conducted properly, informed consent *informs* you of the risks and benefits of a procedure; based on this knowledge you *consent* (or refuse) to go forward. The process should be thorough, unhurried, and tailored to be understood by medical and nonmedical people alike.

Before informed consent can be obtained, the doctor must explain ...

- The nature of the treatment, that is, a description of the proposed treatment or procedure in terms you can understand.
- The benefits, risks, and side effects associated with the procedure or surgery and the risks of not treating the ailment.
- Any alternative treatments, and the risks and benefits of those treatments.
- The probability of success, including an explanation as to how "success" is defined.

Informed Consent Forms

In a recent study of informed consent forms used by 157 hospitals nationwide, only 26 percent contained all four basic informed consent elements, 35 percent included three of the four, and 23 percent contained two of the four[2].

All patients are entitled to informed consent, including the disabled and people who don't speak English. As the patient's bill of rights makes clear, hospitals must make accommodations for these patients, including sign language interpreters for the deaf and translators for the non-English speaking.

Informed Consent and Malpractice

Worried that signing an informed consent form might interfere with your ability to sue if you are the victim of malpractice? Informed consent, performed properly, should make you much more aware of the risks of the procedure for which you have consented, and, by extension, less likely to succeed should you try to sue based on the claim that you "weren't informed" or "didn't know" about a bad outcome. A "bad outcome" that occurs in the course of a properly performed procedure, however, is completely different from a bad outcome that occurs as a result of malpractice. Chapter 20 will help you understand the difference, and how to recognize when malpractice occurs.

If you do sign a consent form, cross out or change sections that you don't understand or which do not reflect your understanding of the risks you are taking or the procedure that is to be done. Be sure to initial any changes made by you to the form.

When Is Informed Consent Required?

As a general rule, regular check-ups or examinations, taking blood pressure, performing x-rays, drawing blood (other than HIV testing), and similar low-risk procedures do not usually require informed consent. Informed consent is generally reserved for: invasive diagnostic and therapeutic procedures (for example, central lines, colonoscopy, and spinal taps) associated with a significant risk of injury or death, administration of anesthesia, and surgical procedures.

When Is Informed Consent Not Necessary?

Informed consent is not necessary ...

+ In an emergency situation (for example, lifesaving emergency surgery on an unconscious patient whose consent is assumed).
+ When the risks are insignificant (for example, getting a chest x-ray).
+ When the patient does not want to know.
+ When the doctor can show that telling the patient will cause psychological harm or upset the patient to the point where a rational decision cannot be made. In this case, the doctor should inform a person selected by the patient to assist the patient in making medical decisions.

Note that *withholding* information—if that's what the patient *wants*—is just as valid a way of respecting a patient's decision-making autonomy as providing them with every last shred of data. A patient who says, "Do whatever you think is right, Doc," has *chosen* to entrust his or her care to the judgment of the doctor. Note also that the doctor's obligation to do no harm (*primum no nocere*) extends to the informed consent process. If providing the details necessary for informed decision making might cause serious emotional distress, that information can be withheld, although it should be provided to a family member or loved one who can then advise the patient.

When Informed Consent Doesn't Count

Informed consent is not valid when the patient is coerced into signing; incapacitated, drunk, or under the influence of drugs; not competent to give consent due to mental impairment; or a minor.

A mentally incapacitated person is "incapable" of giving consent when he or she cannot understand the consequences of his or her own decisions. A man with paranoid delusions who believes the surgeon slated to do his appendectomy is part of an FBI conspiracy to kill him, for example, "lacks capacity" and can be treated against his will. Usually, family members will be relied upon to give consent for incapacitated relatives.

Exercise Your Rights!

Exercise the rights that have been granted to you by law! Inform yourself about your condition, ask lots of questions, and participate in your care. You will help assure that your hospital stay is shorter and safer and that you are better when you go home.

Following are some good questions and suggestions for your doctor concerning *informed consent and patients' rights:*

+ What is my illness or condition?
+ What will happen during the treatment or procedure that is planned for me?
+ What is the likely outcome if I decide not to be treated?
+ What are the benefits of the treatment or procedure?
+ What are the risks and side effects? What is the probability of them happening?
+ Who will perform the procedure or treatment? How many times has this person done this type of treatment or procedure, and what is his or her success rate? I prefer that this treatment or procedure be performed by an experienced doctor.
+ What is the probability that the treatment or procedure will be successful?
+ Are there any alternative treatments and what are their risks and benefits?

Chapter 6

You're In! Now What?

You sat in the emergency room waiting area for five hours, you were on a gurney in the emergency room hallway for another four hours, and you've been examined by two, and possibly quite a few more, doctors. You've been stabbed, poked, and prodded, and, in a fitful hour of sleep, you showed off the part of your posterior that your gown didn't quite cover to dozens (and possibly hundreds) of hospital patients, staff, and visitors. You signed a half-dozen forms, an orderly shuffled you onto the elevator in a wheelchair, and you're finally in your room. What's next?

This chapter introduces the basics of your hospital stay: your room and its amenities (phone and TV), the (notoriously bad) food, typical visiting hours and rules, and other basic elements. The hospital, like any other institution, has its rhythms, and you will be a better participant in your care if you know what to expect and when to expect it.

Hospital Basics #1: Your Room

A hospital room that is clean and pleasant is a harbinger of quality care to come. Your room will not be palatial, but it should be comfortable and clean—especially clean—and if it is not, the nursing supervisor or a patient representative should be notified immediately. You will have a single bed with an adjustable head and foot, with controls that are easily operated. If you have a roommate (or roommates), there should be a curtain that can be drawn for privacy, and these curtains also should be clean. The bathroom, which will be simple and functional, with grab bars next to the toilet and in the shower, also must be clean. Cleanliness is not only each patient's right regarding his or her hospital surroundings, but also critical to patient safety. A clean hospital has less risk of spreading *hospital-acquired* (nosocomial) *infections* that can be among the most devastating complications of a hospital stay (see Chapter 17). Your room *must* be clean; if it is not, insist that it be cleaned or that you be moved to alternate quarters.

Close Quarters

One of the most common concerns expressed by patients regarding roommates is exposure to infectious disease. Those patients who do have potentially communicable illness, however, are placed in isolation rooms (see the "Isolation" description that follows) to minimize the risk of spread. Exposure to HIV is another source of concern; fortunately, the infection is not transmitted by sharing living quarters.

Here's a list of available rooms:

♦ **Private/semi-private.** Rooms in general medical and surgical wards are usually two-bedded, or *semi-private*. Unless there is a particular medical reason for you to be in one, a private room is certain to come at a premium, and your insurance company will insist on your paying some or all of the $100 (or more) per day surcharge. Although the comforts of a private room are obvious, there are few if any medical concerns about sharing a room, and most people adjust to the arrangement without difficulty, often forming friendships with roommates that seem to help with the stress of being in the hospital.

Luxury hospitals, a recent phenomenon, provide *every* patient with a private room. These facilities, usually specialty hospitals (or general hospitals which have set-aside luxury wards), charge several hundred extra dollars a day to provide their patients with all the perks, from private rooms to gourmet meals and quarters for family members.

- **Ward.** Many older hospitals have four or more bedded rooms, or *wards*. As new hospitals are being built and old ones knocked down, this is becoming increasingly rare, and you will be unlikely to find hospitals built after 1960 with multi-bed wards.

- **Isolation.** An isolation room is a private room that you get whether you like it or not. People are put into isolation because they have (or might have) a contagious infectious disease, such as tuberculosis, that might spread to other patients and staff. Visitors and staff have to don masks, gowns, and gloves before entering.

  If you have a loved one in an isolation room, this will clearly be posted on the door. Make sure to stop at the nurse's station to ask about required protective gear *before* entering.

  If you are placed in an isolation room, make sure to ask whether you might have an infectious disease that might have spread to your family or loved ones and whether they should be seen by a doctor to make sure they are not sick.

Isolation Can Save Lives

New York City saw a mini-tuberculosis epidemic in the early 1990s. Aggressive identification of suspected cases, isolation, and treatment of patients—some mandated to take medications against their will—resulted in a marked decline in the incidence of the disease.

- **ICU/CCU (intensive care unit/cardiac care unit).** See Chapter 13.
- **Recovery room.** See Chapter 12.

Television and a Phone

In addition to the room itself are amenities such as the TV and phone. Generally speaking, those *are* the amenities, and both cost money. TVs, mounted to the wall, at the foot of the bed, or extending cranelike on a metal arm, generally run about $5 a day. Unless you are in a private room, you will have a small, handheld speaker connected to the TV by a cable so you may listen without disturbing your roommate. Phones also cost money, though incoming calls are usually free.

There will be a call-bell at your bedside—make sure that your nurse orients you to its use on your arrival. A metal panel on the wall has outlets for oxygen and suction apparatus; in the ICU/CCU there is also a bank of electronic monitors for your bodily functions. Most rooms have a locker (I recommend you send any valuables home with a friend or relative as soon as you are admitted, or, alternatively, ask that they be stored by the hospital for safekeeping), a bedside table with drawers, and an adjustable tray table. There might be a print or two on the wall, and that's about it, except, of course, for the food.

Three Not-So-Hots and a Cot: Hospital Food

Not only are hospitals not known for their food, but, notoriously, they are known for *lousy* food (with the exception of luxury hospitals, which make gourmet food a main attraction for their high-paying clientele). To be fair, hospital food has improved of late, and it is certainly no worse than that to be found in many cafeterias.

Still, the hospital experience is not one that promotes the enjoyment of a meal. Patients, who are sick, are often disinterested in eating. Even those patients who *are* interested in eating might be away from their beds getting a diagnostic procedure (like a chest x-ray) when the food arrives or forbidden to eat by their doctors. By the time they have a chance to get down to it, the food is cold and congealed. And even in the best of circumstances, hospital food is—in a word—*healthful*. Lots of green beans, iceberg lettuce, and boiled, skinless chicken, and not much salt, fat, or sugar. This isn't to say that healthy is *bad,* just that the average American Diabetic Association meal prepared in a hospital kitchen will probably not be as palatable as the same meal prepared in one's own kitchen. Let's just say that if it is the food that is the worst aspect of your hospital stay, you will have had an excellent and complication-free hospitalization.

Your Daily Schedule: Rounds, Tests, and X-Rays

Rounds are conducted by doctors and nurses several times each day. Schedules vary from hospital to hospital, so it is best to ask about the routines in your particular institution. Rounds are the best time to ask questions, especially of your doctor, so find out when you can expect to see them, sit 'em down at your bedside, and ask away. If they're in a rush or give you answers you don't understand, politely remind them that asking questions and getting satisfactory answers is a right guaranteed you by law. Most doctors *prefer* well-informed patients, so your eagerness should be well received. If it isn't, complain to the patient representative or, if you have to, right up the chain of command to the hospital's CEO.

In general, nursing coverage for medical and surgical wards is provided in three eight-hour shifts a day (in the ICU/CCU, nurses might work twelve-hour shifts); nurses conduct their rounds as each shift ends and the next begins. Nurses are an excellent source of information—many maintain that nurses have better people skills, are more patient, and are a better source of information than doctors. Patient education is a central objective of nursing, so you should pick your nurse's brain whenever possible.

And While You're Asleep

Many doctors, especially surgeons, conduct their rounds very early in the morning, while you may still be sleeping. You may even be sleeping in the middle of the day. Either way, your doctors may pass you by without waking you, especially if you are stable and they are in a rush. Rounds are a good time to ask questions, so make sure to *ask* them to wake you!

Diagnostic procedures such as CAT scans, x-rays, and nuclear medicine scans (see Chapter 8) tend to happen in the middle of the day, when the hospital is up and running. Blood drawing is done early—at 5:30 or 6 in the morning—so results will be ready by midday, so *expect* to be awakened by a needle stick. If you are very sick, you will undergo procedures at all hours, so don't be surprised if you are taken for a CAT scan in the middle of the night. The hospital might be busiest during the day, but it is a 24-hours-a-day, 7-days-a-week operation.

Breakfast, lunch, and dinner happen at standard times. Visiting hours tend to run from the early afternoon to the late evening, though this is variable, and the ICU/CCU will be more restrictive and limit the number of people allowed at the bedside at any given time. Children are allowed, though it is unwise to bring very young children onto a busy adult medical ward where there might be an infectious disease risk to their still developing immune systems.

You have a room, a bed, a roommate, a TV, and a phone. Shortly, you will meet the doctors, nurses, technicians, dieticians, housekeeping, and other staff who will participate in your care. Each of these members of your healthcare team has a specific job and routine; Chapter 7 will tell you all about them.

Following are some good questions and suggestions for your doctor concerning *your room and the hospital schedule:*

- ♦ Will I be in a private room, or will I have a roommate?
- ♦ How much does it cost to rent a TV and a phone?
- ♦ Am I at any risk for exposure to infectious disease by having a roommate?
- ♦ Will I be in an isolation room? If so, why? Do I have a communicable disease? Is this a risk to my family?
- ♦ When can I expect to have my blood drawn?
- ♦ When will you or the doctors who are caring for me conduct their rounds? When will they be available to answer questions?
- ♦ When will the nurses be conducting their rounds? Who is the head nurse?

Chapter 7

Doctors and Nurses and Techs, Oh My!: Your Friendly Hospital Staff

Many people will participate in your hospital stay, from the doctor who admitted you to the engineering and maintenance staff who make sure the equipment used in your care functions properly. You will have the most interaction with clinical staff, the people who provide hands-on care, from doctors and nurses to technicians and therapists. This chapter examines the roles of the various clinicians involved in your care. All the better for you to join in to help them get you better.

Your Medical Staff

Most people who are admitted to the hospital are cared for by several doctors; those with complicated problems might be attended by dozens. How do you make sense of this crowd, and who's the boss? Easy. The boss, the one doctor who all others must answer to, is your attending doctor.

Your Attending Doctor

Your attending doctor bears ultimate medical, legal, and moral responsibility for your care. He or she might be your primary care doctor (provided he or she has admitting privileges at your hospital—see Chapter 2), or, if you don't have a primary care doctor, a senior doctor who is assigned to you after you are admitted. If you have a problem that is beyond your primary care doctor's expertise, you might be transferred—with your permission—to the care of another, more experienced attending. Your attending might also transfer you to a *hospitalist,* a physician specializing in the care of hospitalized patients.

In all but the most straightforward of admissions, your attending will need other doctors to assist in your care. If you are admitted with fluid in your lung, for example, your attending might request the assistance of a pulmonary (lung) specialist to help make a diagnosis and guide treatment, but all *decisions* will be made by you and your attending. Such specialists and sub specialists, which cross the spectrum of medical and surgical specialties, are called *consultants.*

Interns, Residents, Fellows, and Medical Students

If you are in a teaching institution (see Chapter 2), you will be cared for by interns, residents, fellows, and medical students. Interns and residents are newly graduated doctors who work for the hospital in *residency* programs, training in areas such as internal medicine (known simply as "medicine"), pediatrics, family practice, and general surgery. It is the intern, ultimately, who gets things done for patients in the hospital, and you are one of thousands who will pass through his or her hands in the course of a very busy year. *Fellows* are doctors who have completed residency and are continuing to train in subspecialty areas (such as gastroenterology, cardiology, and pulmonary medicine).

Interns and residents are incredibly busy and work notoriously long shifts. Typically, a medical intern's day starts at 6:30 or 7 A.M. and ends when the work is done. Mornings are spent presenting newly admitted patients to the supervising attending, while "rounds" are devoted to those already admitted. If you are a "service" patient, that is, if you have been admitted through the emergency room and are being attended by a member of the hospital's staff rather than your own doctor, attending, interns, residents, and medical students will descend on your bedside in one big pack. If your attending is your own doctor, "rounds" will likely precede office hours in the early morning, or follow them in the early evening, and are more likely to be conducted solo. Make sure to ask your doctors when you might expect to see them, as this is the best time for you, your relatives, and loved ones to ask questions.

Typically, interns and residents admit patients when they are *on-call,* a shift that can last anywhere from 24 to 36 or more hours. In busy hospitals, it is not unusual for an intern to admit 20 or more patients in a single on-call shift.

A Hard Day's Night

New York is the only state to restrict the hours of interns and residents. The so-called 405 law dictates that they may work no more than 24 hours in a single shift and 80 hours in a week. Unfortunately, these restrictions are widely ignored, and there are no formal restrictions in the other 49 states.

In other words, your intern and resident are *very* pressed for time. Still, you will spend lots of time with them, and they are an excellent source of information. Bear in mind that they might be in a state of exhaustion when called upon to perform a procedure like a spinal tap (*lumbar puncture*) or central line, and it is your right to refuse the procedure if you feel fatigue might interfere with its proper performance. Twenty-four hours seems a reasonable cut-off; if your intern has been working for longer, insist that you be seen by a better-rested doctor.

Some patients object to being cared for by doctors-in-training, citing their inexperience and refusing to be "experimented on" by house staff. Although this objection is understandable, the care provided in teaching institutions is often better than that in community hospitals, where lack of volume might erode a treating doctor's skills. Further, heightened vigilance about the possibility of medical errors has resulted in increased behind-the-scenes supervision of resident staff. Still, it is your right to insist that your care be provided by more senior members of the hospital staff or by your attending. It is also your right to ask *anyone* who arrives at your bedside to perform a given procedure how many times he or she has performed it in the past and, if they seem unqualified, to insist on a more experienced practitioner.

Medical students spend much of their third and fourth years rotating through teaching hospitals and might also be members of the team providing your care. Sometimes they are the only people who have enough time to sit down and explain your condition in detail. Remember, students *must* ask your permission before interviewing or examining you.

Although some patients may feel annoyed by the constant barrage of questions and examinations that the team approach creates, such redundancy is central to making an accurate diagnosis, choosing the right treatment, and preventing mistakes in your care.

State Licensure and Board Certification

All medical school graduates must take and pass Steps 1 and 2 of the *United States Medical Licensing Exam* (USMLE), co-administered by the *National Board of Medical Examiners* (NBME) and the *Federation of State Medical Boards* (FSMB), prior to beginning internship. Step 3, administered on completion of the internship year, is required to obtain a license to independently practice medicine. Most doctors also take qualifying exams after residency to become *board certified* in their specialty areas. These exams, which are administered by national certifying organizations, are designed to assure competence in the specialties and must be retaken every 7 to 10 years to retain certified status.

If you want to know whether your doctor is board certified, ask him or her directly or visit the American Board of Medical Specialties website at www.abms.org for links to the board certifying agencies for the majority of medical, surgical, and subspecialty areas (see the following list). Each website will allow you to check, by name, the certification status your doctor (board certified doctors are called *diplomats*).

Medical, surgical, and subspecialty board certifying agencies listed with the American Board of Medical Subspecialties include the following:

+ **Medical:** Internal Medicine (including Cardiovascular Disease, Endocrinology, Diabetes, Metabolism, Gastroenterology, Hematology, Infectious Disease, Medical Oncology, Nephrology, Pulmonary Disease, Geriatric Medicine, Critical Care Medicine, Interventional Cardiology, and Sports Medicine), Family Practice, Pediatrics, Emergency Medicine, Psychiatry, Neurology, Dermatology, Physical Medicine and Rehabilitation, Anesthesiology, Preventive Medicine, and Medical Genetics.
+ **Surgical:** General Surgery, Obstetrics and Gynecology, Orthopedic Surgery, Vascular Surgery, Colorectal Surgery, Plastic Surgery, Neurological Surgery, Thoracic Surgery, and Urology.
+ **Diagnostic:** Radiology, Nuclear Medicine, and Pathology.

Visit the MetroMedicine website at www.metromedicine. com/specialtyboards.htm, for a list of qualifying requirements and duration of board certification for a variety of primary care and specialty practitioners.

Surgeons

In contrast to primary care doctors, who attend their patients' medical needs over the long term, surgeons meet many of their patients within hours of operating on them, and follow up only until their wounds are healed. Surgeons, like their medical colleagues, take a team approach to patient care, and will almost always request the input of medical consultants before operating on patients with chronic illnesses such as diabetes or heart disease that might cause complications in the operating room (see Chapter 12 for more information on surgeons and anesthesiologists).

Residency programs in surgery are infamous for their heavy workload, strict hierarchy, and long hours. General surgical residencies last 5 years; high-powered sub-specialists such as pediatric cardiothoracic surgeons might train for 10 or more years after graduating from medical school.

Physician Assistants

Physician assistants are licensed to practice medicine with physician supervision. PAs conduct physical exams, diagnose and treat illnesses, order and interpret tests, counsel on preventive health care, assist in surgery, and in most states can write prescriptions. PA programs are 24 to 25 months long and require two years of college and some experience in health care for admission. Master's degrees are also awarded.

Your Nursing Staff

Your registered nurse (R.N.) might be the graduate of a two- or four-year nursing program. Two-year graduates hold an associate's degree in nursing, and four-year graduates a bachelor of science in nursing (BSN). Both must pass a state qualifying exam to obtain a license to practice nursing.

Your R.N. is not merely the passive receptacle of orders issued by your doctor. He or she is charged with independently assessing and treating patients, educating them about disease and health maintenance, and notifying doctors of changes in patients' status and needed therapy. Although R.N.s cannot write medication orders, they are responsible for assuring that orders and medications administered are safe and appropriate. Nurses *must* follow appropriate patient care orders issued by doctors, but staff nurses answer to senior nursing administrators, not physicians.

We Need Nurses

Why is there such a shortage of nurses in America (see Chapter 3)? Core nursing principles, which emphasize teaching, patient self-advocacy, and diagnosing and treating each patient's *response* to illness, are undervalued in this country, both in terms of the prestige afforded nurses and the amount of money they are paid. How to solve this problem? Increase nurses' pay and recognize nursing as a valuable and highly necessary element of patient care.

The following are other types of nursing practice ...

◆ *Nurse specialists* are R.N.s who have received additional training in the care of patients with specific diseases, such as diabetes, HIV, and stroke, and focus their practice in these areas.

◆ *Nurse practitioners* are R.N.s who have obtained Master's degrees in nursing and are qualified to see patients, establish diagnostic and treatment plans, and prescribe medications under the supervision of a physician. Nurse practitioners often specialize in areas such as geriatrics, family practice, and pediatrics.

◆ *Licensed practical nurses* (L.P.N.s) receive one year of training and provide basic bedside care such as feeding, cleaning, and changing patients, dressing wounds, and measuring blood pressure, pulse, and respirations. They also provide many services traditionally assumed by R.N.s, including administering medications, injections, and starting IV lines. Unlike registered nurses, licensed practical nurses cannot independently assess or treat patients and by law must be under the supervision of an R.N. or a doctor.

◆ *Patient care technicians* (PCTs, nursing aides, or nursing attendants) have less training than L.P.N.s and assist patients with personal care and hygiene, take EKGs, put in IVs, and draw blood. Like L.P.N.s, PCTs must be under the supervision of an R.N. or doctor.

Your nurse is likely to have an associate or bachelor's degree in nursing, though much of your care might be conducted by an L.P.N. or PCT. He or she is responsible for assessing your needs and intervening on your behalf, be it by suggesting needed changes in therapy to your doctor, teaching you about your illness, or providing hands-on treatment such as wound care or IV infusion. You will spend more time with your nurse than any other practitioner during your hospital stay, and you should establish the same kind of collaborative and mutually respectful relationship that you have with your M.D.

If you have difficulties with your nurse, stand up for your rights as a patient in a firm and respectful manner. You are entitled to insist that your medications and treatments be administered on time, that questionable orders be reconfirmed with your doctor, to refuse medication you don't want to take, and to have your pain and other discomfort attended promptly. If you feel that your nurse has not responded appropriately, bring your complaint to the nursing supervisor (*nursing care coordinator*, NCC) or patient representative.

Respect is a valued commodity in the hospital setting. Patients who respond to the stress of illness by making a scene will get attention, at least in the short term, but might wind up being labeled as "verbally abusive" and cause staff to keep their distance. In the long run, patients who stand up for their rights with respect get the best treatment from hospital staff.

Get to Know Your Caretakers

Ask their names, offer a greeting, and grant your nurse and other caretakers the same basic civility you expect for yourself. For better or worse, you are only one of thousands who will cycle through the hospital every year. Straightforward, polite self-advocacy and respect for others, even when you are registering a complaint, is not only good policy in *all* aspects of life, but will help you stand out from the hospital crowd and prompt the staff to go the extra mile in your care.

Pharmacists, Therapists, and Technical Staff

The following sections provide more information on some other individuals you might encounter during your stay at a hospital.

Pharmacists

Pharmacists, like nurses, are not merely the passive receptacles of doctors' orders, but independent practitioners, responsible for assuring the medications they dispense are appropriate for patients and will cause no harm. Pharmacists check for allergies and drug interactions, assure that doses are correct, and suggest substitutions or changes in medication regimens. Increasingly, pharmacists are using computerized systems to check medication orders and assure their safety. Degrees offered in pharmacy include a Doctor of Pharmacy (Pharm.D.), requiring two years of college and four years at a school of pharmacy, and a bachelor of science in pharmacy requiring five years of study. Pharmacists undergo a residency in pharmacy after completion of pharmacy school, take a national licensing exam, and are registered (or licensed) by individual states as *registered pharmacists* (R.Ph.). Visit the American Pharmaceutical Association website at www.aphanet.org for more information on the role of pharmacists and new technologies that help assure medication safety.

Physical Therapists

Physical therapists (PTs) attend conditions affecting movement and coordination and help people debilitated by prolonged hospitalization or illness to regain function. Physical therapists might have a baccalaureate, Master's, or Ph.D. degree and must pass a state administered national exam. For more information on the role of physical therapists, visit the American Physical Therapy Association website at www.apta.org.

Occupational Therapists

Occupational therapists help disabled people with day-to-day activities such as dressing, cooking, bathing, using utensils, transportation, and so on. Where a physical therapist helps people relearn *motor* skills such as walking, an occupational therapist helps them with the tasks they need to function at home or go back to work. Degrees in occupational therapy are offered at the baccalaureate, Master's, and doctorate level, and all occupational therapists take a national certification exam and are licensed by the states. For more information on occupational therapy, visit the American Occupational Therapy Association website at www.aota.com.

Respiratory Therapists

Respiratory therapists (RTs) specialize in the care of patients with lung diseases. RTs administer medications, especially inhaled medicines for conditions such as asthma and emphysema. They also operate respirators, collect arterial blood to measure its oxygen and carbon dioxide content (see Chapter 9), collect sputum for lab testing, care for *tracheostomies* (holes surgeons cut in patients' necks that lead to their windpipes) and perform *pulmonary function testing* (see Chapter 9). Respiratory therapists, who are licensed by the state, work under the supervision of doctors and are required to complete either a two-year associate's degree or a four-year baccalaureate degree.

Nutritionists/Dieticians

Nutritionists specialize in the treatment and prevention of disease through diet. Diet is critical not only in the prevention and management of diabetes and heart disease, but it is also an essential element in the treatment of renal and gastrointestinal disease, and other illnesses. Dieticians teach patients about healthy eating and weight loss; recommend calorie, vitamin, and mineral supplements for wound healing; assist people with weight gain; and design diets for tube feeding. Dieticians are trained at the baccalaureate or Master's level and take a national certification examination. States also regulate dietitians and nutritionists. Visit the Dietician/Nutritionist page of the American Medical Association website at www.ama-assn.org/ama/pub/printcat/4235.html for more information.

Imaging Technicians

These folks take your x-rays, CT scans, ultrasounds, and other imaging studies (see Chapter 9 for more information on imaging modalities). Training levels and requirements for state licensure vary from state to state.

Social Workers

At one time, social workers worked one-on-one with patients to help them deal with alcoholism and substance abuse, psychiatric illness, homelessness, and other social problems. Modern day social workers are much more concerned with obtaining concrete services for patients, such as placing them in shelters, nursing homes, physical rehabilitation facilities, and drug and alcohol treatment centers. Social workers, who are licensed by the state, have baccalaureate and higher degrees and different levels of certification. See the National Association of Social Workers website at www.socialworkers.org for more information.

Patient Representatives

The patient representative is responsible for responding to patient complaints. State and national regulatory and oversight authorities take complaints very seriously, and hospitals are increasingly being required to formally investigate and follow-up in writing any complaint lodged by a patient. Patient representatives might also counsel patients who are refusing to comply with care, explaining why physicians' recommendations are in their best interest.

Administrators-on-Duty (AOD)

The AOD is the after-hours hospital troubleshooter. When a nurse calls in sick, a room is flooded, or a patient wants to register a complaint, it is the AOD who is responsible for fixing the problem if it cannot wait until morning.

Risk Management

This is also known as the legal department. The hospital's lawyers are primarily interested in preventing the hospital from being sued. Although they do not usually interact directly with patients, they can be very effective when it comes to making a complaint. If you're not getting the service you need, merely ask the operator to connect you to risk management, and when you have a lawyer on the phone tell them your *next* call will be to the state department of health.

Housekeeping, Transportation, and Dietary

A great deal of your comfort in the hospital will depend on the unheralded staff whose responsibility it is to assure that your surroundings are clean, your food is hot, and your trips for tests and procedures are conducted promptly, comfortably, and with a modicum of privacy. Housekeepers, transporters, and dietary aides are due the same respect granted the professional staff, and can be a reassuring source of human kindness during an anxiety-filled hospital stay.

Volunteers

Want some company, need someone to buy a newspaper or pick up a paperback for you from the patient library? Call the volunteer department and ask them to send someone around. They should be glad to help.

Following are some good questions and suggestions for your doctor concerning *your hospital staff*:

The following questions apply to your doctor:

+ Will you (my primary care doctor) be my attending doctor in the hospital? If not, who will be my attending doctor?
+ Are you or my attending doctor board certified? In what area?
+ Will my attending doctor see me every day? At what time?
+ When is the best time for me or my relatives to ask my attending doctor questions?
+ Will consultants be called in to help with my care? In what specialties? What will they do? Please notify me of any recommendations they make.
+ Will residents, interns, or medical students be involved in my care?
+ Are volunteers available at this hospital?

These questions are for your nurse:

+ Are you an R.N. or an L.P.N.?
+ How many patients are you caring for?
+ When is the best time to ask you questions?

Chapter 8

Your Daily Schedule, Part One: Making the Diagnosis

You've been admitted, you're in your room, you've met your doctors and nurses. Now it's time to find out what's wrong. You came to the hospital for a reason, right? Kidney stones? A spot on your chest x-ray? A bug in your lung? Whatever the problem, you were admitted so the doctors could *do* something, both to find out what's wrong and to get you better. This chapter focuses on the diagnostic process, especially the tests you will undergo now that you are admitted.

Hurry Up and Wait

Expect to spend a lot of time doing nothing in the hospital. Even the sickest patients spend hours and hours waiting for diagnostic tests and treatments, so don't be surprised if it seems like days have passed and little has happened (especially if you are receiving intravenous medications that are given only once daily). In the hospital, waiting is the name of the game.

Making the Diagnosis, Part One: Blood Tests

Blood tests are a routine part of hospital practice. Expect that you will have many, that they will be repeated during the course of your stay, and that the *phlebotomist* (blood drawer) will arrive at your bedside at 6 A.M., or possibly even earlier, so your results will be ready by midday. Ask about the blood tests that are not described here, and tell your doctor that you want the minimum necessary to properly conduct your care. Multiple blood tests over the course of a long stay can add up enough to enough blood loss to make you anemic[1].

Of the hundreds of blood tests available, you doctor is almost certain to order a *CBC, SMA-7, LFTs,* and a *coagulation profile.*

Complete blood count (CBC) measures the number, shape, and size of *red blood cells* (RBCs), *white blood cells* (WBCs), and *platelets.* RBCs carry oxygen to the tissues of the body and might be high (*polycythemia*), or, more commonly, low (*anemia*). Anemia is *very* common in hospitalized patients, with blood loss and dietary deficiencies of *folate* (*folic acid,* a B vitamin) and iron being the most frequent causes. White cells fight infection; an elevated count (more than 10,000, *leukocytosis*) is common in bacterial infections, and a low count (less than 3,000 to 4,000) is a sign of a depressed immune system. Platelets help blood clot. Low counts, which might lead to spontaneous bleeding, are often found in alcoholics and people with depressed immune systems.

SMA-7 (smack, Chem 7, electrolytes, 'lytes, chemistries) measures sodium (Na), potassium (K), chloride (Cl), bicarbonate (HCO_3), blood urea nitrogen (BUN), creatinine (Cr), and glucose, with calcium (Ca) added to make a "SMA-7 with calcium." This test provides a huge amount of information about a broad spectrum of medical problems, including diabetes, abnormal kidney function, and dehydration.

Liver Function Tests (*LFTs, hepatic profile*) include *SGOT* and *SGPT* (also called *liver enzymes* or *transaminases*), and *bilirubin.* LFT abnormalities are common in hepatitis, gallstones, cirrhosis, alcoholism, and many other conditions. Bilirubin gives urine and stool its brown color; elevated levels (greater than 4 or 5) cause a orange-brown hue to the skin and eyes called jaundice (*icterus*). (A skilled doctor can detect jaundice at bilirubin levels of only 2 or 3.)

Clotting function (*coagulation profile, coags, PT, PTT*) tests the ability of blood to clot. Abnormalities are common in liver disease, shock, and many other conditions.

Specialized Blood Tests

More specialized blood tests, ordered depending on what's wrong with you, include the following:

- Minerals and enzymes such as calcium, phosphate, and LDH
- Hormones such as cortisol, testosterone, and prolactin
- Cholesterol (HDL and LDL) and fats (triglycerides)
- Drug such as Dilantin for epilepsy, digoxin for heart disease, and potentially toxic antibiotics such as gentamicin and vancomycin
- Toxins such as alcohol, cocaine, and other illicit drugs
- Antibodies against infections and diseases such as HIV, hepatitis, syphilis (VDRL or RPR), *systemic lupus erythematosis* (SLE, "lupus"), and rheumatoid arthritis
- Cultures to test for blood-borne infections
- Tumor markers for certain types of cancer
- Arterial blood (*arterial blood gases*, ABGs) for oxygen and carbon dioxide content

---

Arterial Blood

Arterial blood is drawn from an artery in the wrist just below the thumb and is especially helpful for measuring oxygen levels in patients who are short of breath. Venous blood, though easier to get, is normally oxygen depleted. "Arterial sticks" *hurt!* Ask you doctor to first inject a tiny amount of *lidocaine* (local anesthetic) to numb the area—this will make the procedure much more comfortable.

Urine Tests

Your doctor will also order urine tests, such as the following:

+ *Urinalysis* (UA) tests for red and white blood cells, crystals, glucose, and other normal and abnormal urine components to help diagnose kidney and bladder infections (*pyelone-phritis* and *cystitis*), kidney stones (*nephrolithiasis*), diabetes, dehydration, and other conditions.
+ *Urine culture* tests for bacteria that cause urinary infections.
+ *Twenty-four-hour urine collection* helps determine the cause of kidney stones and assesses kidney failure from conditions such as diabetes and high blood pressure (*renal insufficiency*).

Cultures

Doctors *culture* blood, urine, sputum, *cerebrospinal fluid* (the fluid bathing the brain and spinal cord), and other body fluids and tissues to diagnose infections. These specimens are incubated with nutrients, and, when an infection is present, colonies of bacteria grow and become visible to the naked eye. These colonies are tested chemically and microscopically to identify the offending bacteria and to determine which antibiotics will best eradicate the infection.

Biopsies

Biopsies are specimens of tissue sent to the lab for testing. Biopsies are obtained at the bedside with a needle (*fine needle aspiration,* FNA) or in the operating room during surgery. Skin, liver, lymph node, and bone marrow biopsies are conducted at the bedside; masses in the abdomen or chest are biopsied in the operating room or by *CT* or *ultrasound guided biopsy.*

Use Local Anesthetics

Bone marrow biopsies *hurt!* But if your doctor is ordering such a specialized test, you most probably require it to make the best diagnosis and treatment available to you. So make sure the *hematologist* (blood specialist) who does the test uses plenty of local anesthetic to make the procedure a bit easier.

Imaging Studies

Imaging studies include the following:

+ **X-rays (radiographs).** An x-ray is a certainty in the hospital. Chest x-rays (CXRs, "chest films") are performed on just about everyone and help doctors diagnose pneumonia, asthma, emphysema (chronic lung disease), congestive heart failure, rib fractures, and many other problems. Abdominal x-rays are a bit outdated, though they can be useful in diagnosing kidney stones, gallstones, and intestinal blockage (*intestinal obstruction*). X-rays are particularly useful for looking at bone problems, including fractures, dislocations, arthritis, cancer, infections (*osteomyelitis*), and other conditions.

Radiation Exposure

Many people worry about radiation exposure from x-rays. A chest x-ray uses 10 to 30 *milliroentgens* (a measure of radiation equal to one-thousandth of a roentgen), the same amount received from natural sources over a period of a month[2]. It would take several thousand total body x-rays to reach a lethal dose of radiation (approximately 600 roentgens)[3].

+ **Contrast x-rays (contrast studies).** Oral or intravenous *dyes* can greatly enhance x-ray pictures. Contrast x-rays include *angiograms*, which outline arteries and veins in suspected blockage; IVPs (*intravenous pyelograms*), for stones and blocked kidneys (*hydronephrosis*); and *barium enema* and *upper GI (small bowel) series* for tumors and inflammation of the large and small intestine. Contrast dyes, which might contain iodine, can cause kidney damage and allergic reactions, especially in patients with shellfish or seafood allergy. Make sure to tell your doctor if you have these allergies!

Angiograms are invasive procedures with potentially dangerous side effects and the risk of bleeding. The much less invasive magnetic resonance angiography is rapidly replacing this technique (both are described in more detail below).

♦ **CT Scan (computed axial tomography, CAT scan).** CT scanning uses x-rays to make terrific cross-sectional pictures (slices) of the body. CT is particularly good at showing masses (for example, abscesses and tumors) and bleeding, and has rapidly become a favorite tool of surgeons (for example, to diagnose appendicitis), replacing many older, more dangerous, and more invasive x-ray techniques. Before insisting that your doctor do a CT scan instead of x-rays, however, remember that a whole-body CT scan delivers as much radiation as 500 chest x-rays, not to mention the much greater cost.

♦ **MRI (magnetic resonance imaging).** MRI uses magnets instead of x-rays and gives even *better* pictures than CT scans. MRI is also very expensive, and your doctor will use routine x-rays or CT first to make your diagnosis if possible. Like CT, MRI is great at finding bleeding and masses; its high resolution pictures also make it ideal for finding smaller and more subtle problems such as bone infections, damaged cartilage in the knees and other joints, slipped discs (*herniated nucleosus pulposis,* HNP), small tumors, swollen lymph nodes (a potential sign of cancer spread), and blocked blood vessels. The dye used with MRI, *gadolinium,* does not affect the kidney and rarely causes side effects or allergy. MRA (*magnetic resonance angiography*) is rapidly replacing conventional contrast angiography and provides terrific images of blood vessels without the use of invasive catheters and contrast dyes. MRCP (*magnetic resonance cholangiopancreatography*), which outlines the gall bladder and bile ducts, is another new MRI technique that has replaced an older invasive technique, ERCP (see below).

Metals and Magnets

Make *sure* to tell your doctor if you have any metal devices such as pins used to repair fractures or artificial joints before you undergo MRI scanning. These can become dislodged by the powerful magnetic field generated by the scanner, leading to severe injuries and even death!

- **PET scan (positron emission tomography).** A new imaging technique, PET scans help distinguish whether a mass is an infection, a tumor, or benign. PET scanning is still experimental and not widely available.
- **Ultrasound.** Ultrasound, which uses sound waves to make pictures, is the most harmless of the imaging techniques. Conditions diagnosed with ultrasound include blockages and stones in the kidneys and gallbladder, cysts (for example, ovarian cysts), heart problems such as congestive heart failure and valve abnormalities (a heart ultrasound is called *echocardiography* or *echo*), and narrowed arteries and veins, especially in the neck (*carotid duplex ultrasound*) and kidney. Ultrasound is also used to check the age and health of fetuses. Ultrasound doesn't give the same image quality as CT or MR scanning, but it is much cheaper and there are no side effects or allergies.
- **CT and ultrasound guided biopsy.** CT or ultrasound can be used to assist needle placement during a biopsy. A small mass in the liver, for example, which might be missed were the needle inserted randomly, can easily be located with CT or ultrasound and precisely targeted.

◆ **Nuclear imaging.** Nuclear imaging uses very small amounts of radioactive substances to produce pictures of the body. The pictures are not nearly as detailed as CT or MRI scans, but the technique is very good at finding *occult* (hidden) problems missed by other modalities. Nuclear images, and their targets, include *gallium* and *bone scans*, for deep-seated infections and tumors of the body and bones, *HIDA scans* for gall stones and tumors of the bile duct, *thyroid scans* for thyroid conditions, and *VQ scans* for blood clots in the lungs (*pulmonary embolus*). Most of these studies take several hours to a day to complete; a gallium scan takes three days. And don't worry about radiation! The amount used is *less* than a routine diagnostic x-ray.

Nonsurgical Invasive Testing

Biopsies are among the invasive studies that might be done at your bedside. Other invasive bedside tests include the following:

◆ **Angiography.** In angiography, a doctor inserts a catheter into a blood vessel (usually the large vein or artery in the upper thigh), feeds it to the area in question, releases dye, and takes x-rays. Angiography is performed under sterile conditions by masked, gloved, and gowned doctors in an operating room, using light sedation (i.e., you will be drowsy or sleeping lightly) and local anesthesia. Side effects include bleeding, infection, dye allergy, and kidney failure.

◆ **Cardiac catheterization (coronary angiography, cardiac cath).** Cardiac catheterization is a kind of angiogram that outlines the arteries of the heart to show narrowing (*stenosis*) that might be the cause of angina or heart attack. Side effects include flushing, a feeling of intense heat, bleeding, infection, heart attack, and abnormal heart beat. *Angioplasty* might be performed simultaneous to cardiac catheterization.

◆ **Paracentesis.** Paracentesis is the removal of fluid from the abdomen with a needle and syringe. Fluid in the abdomen (*ascites*) is *always* abnormal and can result from cirrhosis of the liver, cancer, tuberculosis, and other conditions. The procedure, which hurts less than it sounds, is performed after careful sterilization of the abdomen with iodine solution and injection of local anesthetic. Side effects include bleeding, infection, and nicking of the intestine (*perforation*) that might require surgical repair.

♦ **Thoracentesis.** Thoracentesis is use of a needle and syringe to remove fluid from around the lungs (*pleural effusion*). Like ascites, a pleural effusion is *always* abnormal; causes include pneumonia, tuberculosis, congestive heart failure, and cancer. The procedure, performed at the lower part of the back of rib cage, is conducted under sterile conditions with local anesthetic. Side effects include bleeding into the chest (*hemothorax*), infection, and a collapsed lung (*pneumothorax*). Hemothorax requires surgery to stop the bleeding; in pneumothorax a large bore *chest tube* is inserted between the ribs into the chest cavity to reinflate the lung.

♦ **Lumbar puncture (LP, spinal tap).** A spinal tap samples the fluid bathing the brain and spinal cord (*cerebrospinal fluid*) to help diagnose bleeding, infection (*meningitis, encephalitis*), and tumors. The procedure, which is conducted while you are in a sitting position or curled on your side in bed, is performed by thoroughly cleansing your lower back with iodine solution and (following an injection of local anesthesia) inserting a long, thin needle into the base of your spine. Done properly, an LP should be *almost* painless. Headache, which can be severe and pounding, is common after LP. Unfortunately, the old rule about staying in a lying position for several hours after an LP to prevent headache has not stood up to close scrutiny; more recent research has focused on the type of needle as most important in preventing headache[4]. Other, rarer side effects include minor bleeding and infection. Blurry vision happens even more rarely, and usually gets better spontaneously[5].

- **Joint Aspiration.** Joint aspiration is the removal of fluid from a swollen joint (*joint effusion*) to diagnose infections and arthritis, including *septic arthritis*, a serious bacterial joint infection. The joint most commonly aspirated is the knee, though orthopedic surgeons will aspirate fluid from any affected joint. The procedure is done under sterile conditions with local anesthesia and might cause bleeding and infection.

- **Endoscopy (colonoscopy and esophagogastroduodeno-scopy, EGD).** Colonoscopy is an excellent means of finding tumors, polyps, inflammation, and other bowel problems. In EGD, a fiber-optic scope is advanced through the mouth, down the esophagus, and into the stomach and small intestine (*duodenum*). Gastric ulcers, duodenal ulcers, and tumors are easily diagnosed by EGD. EGD can cause gagging and is unpleasant, but it should not be painful. Side effects are rare and include rupture of the stomach or intestines (*perforation*) and bleeding—which might require emergency surgery—and infection.

- **Bronchoscopy.** Bronchoscopy uses a fiber-optic scope to explore and biopsy the lungs in persistent and refractory pneumonia, masses, and other lung problems. The procedure is usually performed with mild sedation and might cause bleeding, infection, and *pneumothorax*.

Other common tests that your doctor might order to help find out what's wrong include:

- **Electrocardiogram (EKG).** An EKG is a paper tracing of the heart's electrical activity and helps diagnose heart attack, narrowed coronary arteries, and abnormal heart rhythm. Every patient will have an EKG on admission to the hospital.

- **Stress testing.** Stress testing uses EKG or nuclear imaging (*thallium*) to measure the heart's response to exercise (*exercise stress testing*) or *dipyridamole* (*Persantine*, a drug that reproduces the effects of exercise on the heart) to diagnose narrowed coronary arteries. Side effects include angina, heart attack, and abnormal heart rhythm, though these are rare.

♦ **Pulmonary function testing (PFTs).** Pulmonary function testing noninvasively measures lung function. The procedure, which involves blowing into a machine, helps diagnose asthma and emphysema, and the response of these diseases to medication. Doctors might also *provoke* asthma (*bronchoprovocation* or *methacholine testing*) during pulmonary function testing as part of a diagnostic work-up. Side effects are rare.

♦ **Electroencephalography (EEG).** EEGs measures brain waves to determine the cause of epilepsy. Dozens of wire leads are affixed to the scalp, and a long, wide paper with tracings on it slides from the side of the machine.

Your doctor will recommend one or several of these common diagnostic procedures while you are in the hospital. If you are in a teaching institution—where the doctors consider a broader spectrum of possibilities for what's wrong with their patients— you will undergo more testing than in a community hospital. It is a rule of thumb that doctors will start out with the simple and noninvasive tests, and if that doesn't lead to a diagnosis, move to the more complicated and invasive tests. If you have a mass in your lung, for example, the doctors will recommend bronchoscopy first, and if that doesn't lead to a diagnosis, an operation to take a biopsy (open lung biopsy).

Many tests require that you eat nothing for breakfast on the day of the exam; in bigger and busier hospitals this can mean a long and hungry wait for a procedure that might be suddenly cancelled if an emergency comes along and bumps you from the schedule. And don't be surprised if you start to feel like a pincushion! Blood tests are a certainty in the hospital, sometimes at the rate of two or three a day, and even more frequently in the ICU. Don't get angry, but don't forget to ask for an explanation of what the tests are for, refuse those for which your doctor has no good explanation, and insist that only the minimum number be done to get you better and *out* of the hospital.

Following are some good questions and suggestions for your doctor concerning *diagnostic testing:*

◆ What diagnostic tests will I undergo in the hospital? What will the results show you? Please notify me of these results!

◆ Will I undergo any dangerous or invasive diagnostic tests? What are the risks of these tests? Are there alternative, safer tests?

◆ Please make sure that I am provided with adequate pain medicine during and after any painful procedures!

◆ Will contrast dye be used on me? If so, is it likely that I will have an allergic reaction or that my kidneys will be damaged?

◆ Please make sure that blood tests are kept to the absolute minimum necessary to care for me!

◆ If I need a blood gas, please provide me with a local anesthetic to make it less painful!

Chapter 9

So What's Wrong with Me, Doc?

The human body is a complicated machine. So much can go wrong with it. The *full* spectrum of diseases is beyond the book's scope, but a few thumbnail sketches of the most prevalent conditions might help further your understanding of your hospital stay.

Common Diseases: A Primer

This short review of common diseases that lead to hospital admission, by no means complete, should give you a head start on better understanding your own medical condition. Hopefully, it will prompt you to find out more by referring to the websites listed in the following sections. As always, this information is intended to help you participate in your care and get out of the hospital faster and in much better shape than when you went in. For information on what your doctor will do once your condition is diagnosed, see Chapter 10.

Gastrointestinal Disease

The gastrointestinal, or GI, tract extends from the mouth to the anus. Along the way, there is the *esophagus* (the swallowing tube that leads from the mouth to the stomach), the stomach, the small intestine (the *duodenum, jejenum,* and *ileum*), and the large intestine (*colon*). The *appendix* is a pinkylike pouch of intestine attached to the colon. The liver, pancreas, and gall bladder are also GI organs. Check out the Directory of Digestive Diseases Organizations For Patients at www.niddk.nih.gov/health/digest/pubs/ddorgpat/ddorgpat.htm for a comprehensive list of patient-friendly organizations and websites for more information on GI diseases.

GI problems are among the most common hospital diagnoses. They include the following:

- **GI bleeding.** GI bleeding from the stomach and small intestine is called "upper" GI bleeding; and that in the large intestine is called "lower" GI bleeding. Vomiting of blood, which can be either bright red or have the appearance of coffee grounds (digested blood), is commonly caused by gastric and duodenal ulcers, tumors, and violent retching (*Mallory-Weiss tear*). Alcoholics with cirrhosis can bleed from ruptured, swollen esophageal blood vessels (*varices*). When bleeding in the stomach or small intestine is particularly brisk, stool turns dark purplish-black (*melena*). Rectal bleeding most commonly results from hemorrhoids, diverticula (see Chapter 4), inflammatory bowel disease (*Crohn's disease* and *ulcerative colitis*, see the last bullet within this list), and tumors. Doctors diagnose GI bleeding by EGD and colonoscopy (see Chapter 8).

- **Liver Disease and Cirrhosis.** Alcohol and hepatitis C are the major causes of liver disease in America. Inflammation of the liver is *hepatitis*, and scarring of the liver is *cirrhosis*. Cirrhosis causes jaundiced skin, a protuberant, fluid filled abdomen (*ascites*), spindly arms and legs, delirium (*hepatic encephalopathy*), GI bleeding, and death.

- **Disease of the Gall Bladder and Bile Duct (*biliary tree*).** Bile, which helps digest food, is produced by the liver, stored in the gall bladder, and secreted through the bile duct into the intestine. A blockage anywhere along the way can cause abdominal pain and jaundice. Common causes of blockage include gallstones (*cholelithiasis*), tumors, and *strictures* (narrowing due to scarring). Doctors diagnose biliary problems with ultrasound, CT scans, and MRCP (see Chapter 8), as well as by using an endoscope to look directly at the bile duct, a procedure whose name, *endoscopic retrograde cholangiopancreatography*, is always abbreviated as ERCP (see Chapter 8).

♦ **Pancreatitis.** Almost always caused by alcohol, pancreatitis (inflammation of the pancreas) is diagnosed by blood tests, ultrasound, CT scan, or ERCP (see Chapter 8).

Your Liver, Biliary Tree, and Pancreas on the Web

Visit the Methodist Health Care System (Houston, Texas) website at www.methodisthealth.com/liver/index.htm for comprehensive, patient-friendly information on diseases, tests, and the anatomy and function of the liver, gallbladder, biliary tree, and pancreas.

♦ **Inflammatory bowel disease (IBD).** *Crohn's disease* and *ulcerative colitis* cause ulceration and bleeding in the large intestine; Crohn's disease might also cause ulcers in the small intestine and open connections between the intestines and skin (*fistulas*). Doctors diagnose IBD with colonoscopy and EGD (see Chapter 8) and treat these conditions with antibiotics and powerful anti-inflammatory agents such as Prednisone. Visit the Crohn's & Colitis Foundation of America, Inc., website at www.ccfa.org for more information on inflammatory bowel disease and its treatment.

Pulmonary (Lung) Disease

Pulmonary disease affects the windpipe (trachea), air passages (bronchi), and lungs, and is especially common in smokers. Pneumonia, asthma, and COPD are the most common pulmonary diseases seen in the hospital.

♦ **Pneumonia.** Pneumonia, an infection of the lungs, is the second most common cause of hospital admission for the elderly, and, along with asthma and bronchitis, the third most common cause of admission for those aged 45 to 64. Doctors diagnose pneumonia by listening for a fine bubbling sound (*rales*) during a lung exam with a stethoscope and by looking at a chest x-ray, which shows a hazy white area (*infiltrate*) where the lung is infected. In severe pneumonia, or pneumonia that is not responding to treatment, bronchoscopy (see Chapter 8) might be necessary to clarify the diagnosis and guide therapy. Pneumonia may be treated in the hospital with intravenous antibiotics, or, if it is not severe, at home with pills.

♦ **Asthma.** Download "Controlling Your Asthma," a brochure issued by the National Heart, Lung, and Blood Institute at www.nhlbi.nih.gov/health/public/lung/asthma/asth_fs.pdf for more information on asthma.

♦ **Chronic obstructive pulmonary disease (COPD).** COPD is most often diagnosed in smokers or ex-smokers. Like asthma, COPD (which includes emphysema and chronic bronchitis) causes inflammation and narrowing of the airways, resulting in wheezing and difficulty breathing. Unlike asthma, COPD causes irreversible damage to the lungs and can leave its victims permanently short of breath. Doctors diagnose COPD by listening for wheezing and reduced air movement during a lung exam, by looking at chest x-rays, and through pulmonary function testing (see Chapter 8), which shows severely reduced flow of air in the lungs. When COPD is severe, home oxygen might be necessary. To prevent COPD, *don't smoke*. Download "Chronic Obstructive Pulmonary disease," published by the National Heart, Lung, and Blood Institute at www.nhlbi.nih.gov/health/public/lung/other/copd/index.htm for comprehensive information on COPD.

The American Lung Association, at www.lungusa.org, is an excellent source of additional information on lung disease.

Cancer

Cancer can affect any organ in the body. Lung cancer is the leading cancer killer of both men and women and a frequent hospital diagnosis. Other common cancers include breast, colon, cervix, and stomach cancer, Hodgkins Disease, lymphoma, and many others. Although a full discussion of cancer is beyond the scope of this book, a few general principles apply to the disease and its treatment. Most important is "stage." Stage, which ranges from 1 to 4 and describes the extent to which a cancer has spread, has an enormous impact on treatment and prognosis (another staging system that your doctor may use is the TNM system). Early stage cancers are small, confined to one area, and tend to be more curable; late stage cancers are more widespread (*metastatic*) and difficult to treat. The underlying health of the affected patient is also critical to treatment and prognosis, as people who are infirm might not be able to withstand the rigors of surgery, chemotherapy, and radiation treatment. When discussing cancer survival, doctors speak of two- and five-year survival rates to describe the percentage of patients who survive for these periods of time. In general, patients who survive five years are considered to be cured from cancer.

Chemotherapy and other cancer treatments are not always intended to cure. Still, "incurable" cancer might respond partially to treatment, and affected patients survive for months or even years longer than they would have without treatment. Surgery, radiation, chemotherapy, and hormonal therapy can also relieve symptoms such as pain and shortness of breath (see Chapter 19 for more information on "noncurative" approaches to terminal illness). Doctors use the spectrum of diagnostic modalities to diagnose cancer and always biopsy a suspicious mass. The American Cancer Society website, www.cancer.org, has more information on cancer, links to support groups, news, and a comprehensive, interactive guide to treatment options and prognosis for virtually every type of cancer (see Chapter 19 for more details on this excellent website).

Infectious Disease

The majority of infections seen in the hospital are caused by viruses; most others are bacterial, with fungal infections and tuberculosis making up a small but significant minority. Most viral infections resolve spontaneously, while bacterial, fungal, and tubercular infections require treatment. The elderly, bed bound, and those with chronic illnesses such as heart disease, diabetes, stroke, and alcoholism are more likely to develop serious bacterial infections, and, because bacteria can rapidly cause death in these groups, doctors will treat them aggressively with intravenous antibiotics, even when infection is only suspected. Similarly, doctors might take a "watchful waiting" approach to those who are younger and healthier, choosing to wait and treat a proven infection rather than use antibiotics unnecessarily. To diagnose infections, doctors look for fever, an *elevated white blood cell count,* and also *culture* blood, urine, and other body fluids (see Chapter 8). Fever is an important sign of infection; the elderly people and those who are critically ill can have a serious infection *without* fever. Patients with depressed immune systems (for example, people with AIDS or those who are being treated with cancer chemotherapy or immune suppressive therapy after an organ transplant) are particularly susceptible to serious and life-threatening infections. Diabetics are prone to repeated infections in their feet and legs, sometimes leading to gangrene and amputation.

Tuberculosis, though relatively rare, continues to be a problem in the United States, especially among alcoholics, the homeless, drug addicts, and those with AIDS. If you have TB, make sure that everyone who has been in close contact with you for the last six months to a year undergoes a PPD to see if they've been infected.

Common infections include the following:

♦ *Pneumonia* (see the preceding "Pulmonary [Lung] Disease" section)

♦ *Meningitis,* an infection, usually bacterial, in the fluid bathing the spinal cord, diagnosed by spinal tap (*lumbar puncture,* Chapters 4 and 8)

- *Encephalitis,* an infection of the brain and spinal cord, usually viral (and usually less dangerous than meningitis), also diagnosed by spinal tap
- *Pyelonephritis* (kidney infection, see Chapter 4)
- *Cellulitis,* an infection of the skin, causing redness, warmth, tenderness, and swelling of the affected area

---

Inflammation

The four essential components of inflammation are swelling, pain, redness, and warmth. In Latin, the root language for many medical terms, these are *tumor, dolor, rubor,* and *calor.*

- *Abscess,* a swollen, tender pus-filled mass
- *Acute gastroenteritis* (AGE), or "stomach flu," causing vomiting, diarrhea, and abdominal pain; usually viral, most AGE resolves without antibiotics
- *Viral syndrome,* a *febrile* illness (an illness with fever), such as a head cold or the flu that clears up on its own

The Infectious Disease Society of California has a patient-friendly question and answer page on infectious disease at www.idac.org (under *patient information*). Virtual Hospital, a service of the University of Iowa at www.vh.org, also has patient-oriented information on infectious diseases (browse by *Topic* under *For Patients,* and click on *infections*).

Renal (Kidney) Disease

Renal failure (end stage renal failure, ESRD) is a condition in which the kidneys are unable to remove toxins and waste from the blood and excrete them in the urine. The most common causes of renal failure in America are high blood pressure and diabetes, and the diligent control of these diseases is critical to preventing renal failure. Other causes of renal failure include inflammation of the kidney (*glomerulonephritis*) from *autoimmune diseases* such as *systemic lupus erythematosis* and toxins (especially medications such as ibuprofen [Motrin], lithium, and others).

Patients with renal failure are treated with *hemodialysis,* in which a machine clears waste from the blood, and *peritoneal dialysis*—which can be done at home—in which fluid is instilled into the abdominal cavity through a catheter and drained back out again. Both treatments require the surgical placement of catheters; in the upper arm for hemodialysis, and in the abdomen for peritoneal dialysis. Both types of catheters can lead to serious infections and must be kept clean. Kidney dysfunction (*azotemia,* or *renal insufficiency*) can also result from severe dehydration; doctors treat this condition with IV fluid to restore blood volume.

For more information on renal failure and kidney disease, the National Institute of Diabetes and Digestive and Kidney Diseases, at www.niddk.nih.gov, has patient-friendly information and brochures, and the National Kidney Foundation, at www. kidney.org also has patient- and family-oriented information.

Stroke and Neurologic Disease

Stroke results from a blocked blood vessel in the brain. Causes include hardening of the arteries (atherosclerosis, also a cause of blocked coronary arteries), blood clots, bleeding in the brain, brain tumors, and, less commonly, a brain abscess. Typical signs of stroke include weakness and/or numbness on one side of the face or body, slurred speech, dizziness and loss of balance, and the inability to speak or understand when spoken to (*aphasia*). Doctors diagnose stroke by these characteristic findings and with CAT scan or MRI of the brain. Untreated or poorly controlled high blood pressure is the most common cause of stroke and recurrent stroke, and long-term aggressive blood pressure control is *essential* to its prevention. People with *atrial fibrillation,* a common type of abnormal heart rhythm (and a frequent cause of palpitations in older people) can develop blood clots in the chambers of the heart (*thrombi*) that can break off and travel to the brain (*emboli*) causing stroke; blood thinners such as heparin and warfarin (Coumadin) help prevent this complication.

Stroke Side Effects

People who have strokes are at very high risk for developing bedsores, contractures (bent, stiff arms and legs), and blood clots in the legs and lungs while they are in the hospital if they do not receive proper nursing care, physical therapy, and blood thinners. The prevention of these complications is one of the most important ways to advocate for a hospitalized loved one (see Chapter 17).

Dementia, with loss of memory, unpredictable mood swings, and inappropriate or uninhibited behavior, can result from medical illness (for example, AIDS, a low functioning thyroid disease, long standing syphilis, and vitamin B_{12} deficiency), depression, or brain diseases such as Alzheimer's. Dementia may also be caused by medications, a particular hazard among elderly people who are often on ten or more medicines simultaneously. So-called *polypharmacy* often results from frequent sub-specialty consultation—each doctor adds a medicine specific to his or her area of expertise. It is the responsibility of the primary care doctor to review the medication list for possible adverse interactions and unnecessary drugs—frequently all that is required to make dementia disappear. Dementia is *not* a normal part of aging, and affected patients, young or old, should be carefully evaluated for a treatable (or preventable) cause.

Neuropathy, pain and numbness in the feet and hands, is especially common in diabetics, and can lead to repeated foot injury and amputation. Alcoholics and people with HIV also get neuropathy.

The American Academy of Neurology has patient-oriented information and testimonials by people with different neurologic illnesses at www.thebrainmatters.org.

Autoimmune Disease

Autoimmune diseases result when the immune system attacks normal body tissues. Rheumatoid arthritis, systemic lupus erythematosis, and Crohn's disease are common autoimmune diseases. Visit the patient information section of the American Autoimmune Related Disease Association, Inc., at www.aarda. org for more information on individual conditions.

Calling for Donors!

Most American hospitals are chronically short of blood. If you are a healthy person, free of infectious disease, your blood is wanted! To find out where to donate in your area, visit the American Red Cross website at www.redcross.org/donate/ donate.html or call 1-800-GIVE-LIFE (1-800-448-3543).

Blood Disease

Anemia, the most common blood disease, is caused by blood loss, iron deficiency, vitamin B_{12} and folate deficiency (especially in alcoholics), and chronic illness. If anemia is severe, with hematocrit less than 15 to 20 percent (the percentage of blood comprised by red blood cells is normally 40 to 45 percent), blood transfusion might be required. Bleeding disorders, in which the failure of blood to clot properly causes spontaneous hemorrhaging into the skin, conjunctiva (lining of the eyes), gums, and body cavities, is commonly seen in blood infection (sepsis), critical illness, cancer, leukemia (cancer of the white blood cells), multi-trauma, and people with cirrhosis. The complete blood count (CBC), clotting profile, and bone marrow biopsy are important diagnostic tools used to investigate blood diseases (see Chapter 8). Visit the hematology division of the Mayo Clinic website at www.mayo.edu for more information on blood diseases, or connect to multiple blood disease related links at the patient group links page of the American Society of Hematology at www.hematology.org. See Chapter 12 for information on transfusion during surgery, including options for blood storage and transfusion-free surgery.

Fluid and Electrolyte Abnormalities

Water and salt (*electrolytes*) are critical components of blood. Too little water and salt (dehydration), and too much water and salt (*fluid overload*), are commonly seen in the hospital. Sodium, potassium, chloride, bicarbonate, calcium, and magnesium are all critical electrolytes that your doctor might want to monitor. Doctors diagnose fluid and electrolyte problems by physical examination and blood tests, especially the SMA-7 (see Chapter 8). Dehydration causes dry mouth, cracked lips, sunken eyes, and reduced urination; fluid overload causes swelling of the ankles, increased urination, and difficulty breathing. Dehydration is treated with IV fluid, and fluid overload is treated with diuretics ("water pills," see Chapter 10). If you are receiving IV fluid for dehydration, make sure your doctor and nurse check you frequently to assure you are not getting too much fluid. Most people can receive 100 cc per hour of IV fluid with little difficulty. Rates as high as 250 cc to 500 cc per hour can lead to fluid build-up in the lungs (pulmonary edema)—especially in elderly people or those with congestive heart failure—serious shortness of breath, and even respiratory failure.

Drug and Alcohol Addiction

Alcohol affects every organ system in the body. Alcoholics are highly susceptible to infections and pneumonia, which can progress and cause death very rapidly; and alcoholic liver disease (cirrhosis) is a common cause of death by gastrointestinal bleeding. Alcoholics are also prone to bleeding ulcers in the stomach and intestine, neuropathy, cancer, and heart disease. Delirium tremens (DTs), which (unpredictably) occur between twenty-four hours and ten days after an alcoholic stops drinking, causes agitation, confusion, combativeness, seizures, and death.

Intravenous drug abuse (IVDA) is the most dangerous form of drug abuse, causing overdose, skin infections (*cellulitis*), abscesses, infection of the heart valves (*endocarditis*), hepatitis B and C, and AIDS. Cocaine abuse can cause death by heart attack. All illicit drug use can lead to *addiction*, a behavioral syndrome characterized by a downward spiral of escalating drug use, deteriorating health, loss of employment and family ties, homelessness, incarceration, and death.

Surgical Conditions

The need for surgery, whether for a ruptured appendix or a tummy tuck, is one of the most common causes for hospital admission. For more information, see Chapter 12.

Following are some good questions and suggestions for your doctor concerning *your medical condition:*

These apply to all medical conditions:

+ What is the name of my medical condition?
+ Please describe my medical condition in plain English.
+ Is my medical condition acute or chronic? What kinds of long-term problems can it cause?
+ Is there an effective treatment for my medical condition? What is it?
+ For how long will I have to take medications or other treatments?
+ Do diet, weight, and exercise habits influence my medical condition?
+ Can I expect to be cured from my medical condition?

These questions apply to cancer:

+ What kind of cancer do I have and what stage is it?
+ Can my cancer be cured?
+ Am I fit enough to withstand cancer treatment?
+ If my cancer cannot be cured, am I a candidate for treatment that will prolong my life and relieve my symptoms?
+ What are the two-year and five-year survival rates for my cancer, both with and without treatment?

These questions apply to stroke:

+ What caused my stroke? Do I need a blood thinner to prevent another stroke?
+ Did high blood pressure, diabetes, or atrial fibrillation cause me to have a stroke? If so, are these conditions

being treated? If I have high blood pressure and diabetes, are they well controlled?

+ Please make sure to provide me (or my loved one) with protection from bedsores, blood clots, and contractures! (An *essential* request!)
+ Please make sure that I (or my loved one) begin physical therapy as soon as possible!

The following apply to kidney disease and renal failure:

+ Are my kidneys failing? How bad are they?
+ Are diabetes or high blood pressure harming my kidneys?
+ Will I need dialysis?
+ Which is better for me: hemodialysis or peritoneal dialysis?

These question apply to lung disease:

+ Is my lung disease chronic, and will it get worse?
+ Would I benefit from oxygen at home?
+ Please show me how to properly use my metered dose inhaler (pump) for asthma, emphysema, or COPD. Please provide me with a spacer.
+ I have pets and carpets at home. Is this affecting my lung disease? Should they be removed?
+ Will you help me stop smoking?

Ask these questions about infectious disease:

+ Do I have a bacterial infection, or is my condition more likely to be viral? Please do not treat me with antibiotics unless it is absolutely necessary!
+ Can my family or loved ones catch my infectious disease? How do I protect them?
+ Do I have tuberculosis, and, if so, should the people who have been in contact with me be screened for this disease?

Ask these questions about blood disease and anemia:

+ What is my hematocrit? Am I anemic? What is the cause of my anemia? How is my anemia treated?

- Do I need a transfusion? What will happen if I refuse transfusion?
- What are the alternatives to transfusion?

Ask these questions about dehydration and fluid therapy:
- How much IV fluid am I receiving? Is that a lot? For how long will I have to receive it? Please make sure to avoid my receiving too much fluid!

Chapter 10

Your Daily Schedule, Part Two: Treatment

Sometimes what your doctors are planning to do to you is obvious. A surgeon prodded your belly in the emergency room, you hit the ceiling, and he told you it was time to part with your appendix. Simple. Other times, things aren't so clear. You noticed a drop of blood in the toilet, so they did a CAT scan. That wasn't enough, so they did a colonoscopy, and now they're rubbing their chins and saying they think it might be your large intestine, but it could also be your pancreas. The best thing would be to put you on some medications and see what happens. Medicine is a science, with a lot of educated guesswork.

This chapter will review some of the common therapies doctors use to treat what ails you, as well as some of the dangers associated with these therapies and how to avoid them, while Chapter 11 will go into more depth on medications. Should you come across a therapy *you* don't know about, *ask* what it is, what it is hoped to accomplish, and what, if any, are its toxicities and side effects.

Common Hospital Therapies: A Primer

If there is a therapy recommended by your doctor that is not mentioned here or that you do not understand, ask for an explanation and make sure that you understand both the benefits and possible side effects before you consent. Most recommended therapies will be to your benefit; more than a few, unfortunately, have side effects you might not want to risk, others might be done as a matter of convenience rather than because they *must* be done to make you better. Remember: *ask, inform* yourself about your care, and *participate* in medical decision making; you'll be a more satisfied patient and get out of the hospital quicker and healthier if you do.

Intravenous Therapy

Just about every hospitalized patient gets an IV. People expect IVs, and that the medicines given through an IV are more powerful and will get them better quicker and out of the hospital sooner than medicines given by mouth. This is true in many cases, but IVs are often unnecessary, and they can cause some very serious problems (see the following list). So if you have an IV, make sure to ask your doctor if you *really* need it. Some of the therapies given IV are as follows:

+ **Fluids.** Fluids are given IV to people who are dehydrated, when they are unable to eat or drink (for example, patients who are on a respirator or who are vomiting), or when they are forbidden to eat or drink. Salt water (*saline*) comprises most IV fluid, usually with some glucose added to maintain blood sugar. Concentrations of saline include 0.9 percent sodium chloride (NaCl), or *normal* saline, and 0.45 percent NaCl, or *half normal* saline. Potassium (K) is commonly added to saline. *Lactated Ringer's* is an IV fluid favored by surgeons.

+ **Antibiotics.** Doctors use IVs to get antibiotics into people's blood stream quickly and in high doses. The most important consideration in deciding to use IV antibiotics includes the type of antibiotic needed—some antibiotics used to treat severe infections can *only* be given IV—and how sick the patient is. An elderly person with heart disease, for example, would need IV antibiotics to rapidly treat an infection and prevent it from getting worse, while a younger person with no chronic illnesses might do very well with a trial of oral antibiotics and close observation.

+ **Medications.** Thousands of medications are given IV. Chapter 11 will review some of the more common medications used in the hospital, including antibiotics.

♦ **Nutrition.** Patients who are unable to eat for long periods of time might be "fed" through an IV (*parenteral nutrition*), although this therapy can have nasty side effects, including burning at the IV site and damage to the surrounding tissue. Reasons for parenteral nutrition include severe pancreatitis (swelling of the pancreas, often due to alcohol abuse), the inability to eat for more than 10 days, nutrient supplementation for very thin (*cachectic*) people before major surgery, and as an aide in wound healing[1].

♦ **Blood transfusion.** You can't get blood without an IV. But make sure you *need* the transfusion before agreeing to it! People who are actively bleeding or have a very low hematocrit (20 percent is the usual cut-off, approximately half normal) are good candidates for transfusion; this number might be a little bit lower in stronger patients who are better able to tolerate severe anemia and higher in those who are old and frail. If your doctor recommends a transfusion for you, ask about your hematocrit and whether the transfusion is *really* necessary. If blood loss has stopped, ask if you might take iron and vitamin supplements to build up your red blood cell count, with close follow-up to make sure your hematocrit is not dropping further. A "'crit" of less than 15 percent, however, can be life threatening, and a transfusion is an absolute necessity. And don't forget to ask your nurse or doctor to make sure the blood is labeled with *your* name and *your* medical record number. Transfusing the wrong blood *happens*, and it can result in serious reactions.

Complications of IVs can be *very* serious. Infections in the skin (*cellulitis* and *abscesses*) at the IV site are common; prevent them by assuring the IV site is cleaned and dressed on a daily basis and that the IV is changed to a different site at least every three days. Blood clots are another problem, especially with central lines, and must be treated with blood thinners (which can themselves be dangerous). Other hazards of central lines include a generalized and potentially fatal blood infection (*sepsis*), bleeding, and collapse of a lung (see also Chapters 1 and 17).

Do You Really Need an IV?

Ask your doctor if you *really* need an IV, whether you might take your antibiotics or other medications by mouth instead, and be *especially* fussy when it comes to central lines. Make sure the IV site is kept clean and dressed on a daily basis and changed every three days, and if the site shows even a hint of redness, swelling, warmth, or tenderness, demand that it be taken out. (If your doctor or nurse doesn't move quickly enough, pull it out yourself and press a gauze or clean towel to the vein for 10 minutes to stop the bleeding.)

Oxygen Therapy

Oxygen is delivered via face mask or through nasal prongs (nasal *cannula*) in liters per minute (range: 2 to 5) or as a percentage of inspired air (range: 30 to 100 percent). Oxygen therapy is used in a variety of medical conditions, and is most useful when blood oxygen levels are low from heart or lung disease such as COPD or congestive heart failure. Your doctor might ask to assess the level in your blood with an *arterial blood gas* (see Chapter 8). Respirators (ventilators) are used for people who can't breathe at all (see Chapter 13).

Take Note!

Oxygen therapy can dangerously slow—and even stop—respirations in people with severe lung disease such as emphysema.

Ostomies and Pegs

Ostomies are surgically created connections between a body cavity and the skin, such as the stomach, small intestine, and large intestine (*gastrostomy, ileostomy, jejenostomy, colostomy*), kidney and bladder (*nephrostomy, cystostomy*), and windpipe (*tracheostomy*). Surgeons perform ostomies when normal pathways are blocked or not functioning. In colon cancer, for example, a part of the rectum might have to be removed, leaving the surgeon no choice but to create a colostomy with the remaining end of the large intestine.

People who are unable to swallow or are in a coma might have a tube placed directly through the abdominal wall into the stomach to allow feeding (*percutaneous endogastric* [PEG], or *gastrostomy* tube [G-tube]). If your doctor recommends that you have a PEG, make *sure* there has been a full assessment of your ability to swallow before consenting to the procedure. If you have an elderly, demented relative who lives in a nursing home, make *double* sure the PEG is necessary. Many nursing home patients *can* eat; unfortunately, the nursing home staff might be unwilling or unable to spend the time necessary to feed their elderly charges by hand.

Nasogastric Tubes

Nasogastric tubes (NG tubes) are long, thin plastic tubes that go from the nose to the stomach. NG tubes are used to check for bleeding in the stomach and to suction out gas and stomach juices when there is blockage of the intestines (*obstruction*). *Feeding tubes* are longer, thinner, and softer than NG tubes, and are used to give people liquid nutrition when they are unable to eat by mouth. Both NG tubes and feeding tubes can cause inhalation of stomach contents (*aspiration*) and a nasty pneumonia, and are a temporary measure only.

If you need an NG tube, be warned! Putting in the tube is unpleasant! Ask your doctor to use topical anesthesia spray to numb your nose and throat beforehand; this will make the procedure *much* more comfortable. The tubes can damage the mucus membranes of the nose and cause bleeding in the stomach and should not be left in place for more than a half hour or so, except in intestinal obstruction. When attached to a suction pump for obstruction, the dial on the pump (which is usually connected to a port in the wall at the head of the bed) must *always* be set at "intermittent" (rather than "continuous") suction to prevent damage to the lining of the stomach.

Foley Catheters

Foley catheters are long, thin plastic catheters that are threaded through the urethra into the bladder, allowing urine to flow into a plastic bag. Foley catheters are used in people who have a blockage of urine flow and are unable to empty their bladders, and to measure the amount of urine people produce in response to IV fluids or medications. Foley catheters are also used to prevent people who can't get out of bed from soiling themselves, although this use is frequently inappropriate and can lead to dangerous bladder infections (see Chapter 17).

Wound Care

Wounds can result from prolonged immobilization (*decubitus ulcers, pressure sores,* or *bedsores*), trauma, surgery, and infections. Wounds are very common in diabetics, who, because of narrowing of blood vessels (*peripheral vascular disease*) and reduced sensation (*neuropathy*), are especially prone to sores and infections of the feet and legs. *Venous stasis disease,* in which the veins in the legs do not function properly, allowing blood to back up and pool in the lower legs, typically causes shallow, dirty ulcers above the ankle on the inside of the leg. Treatment includes scraping out infected material (*debridement*), frequent dressing changes, and, when all else fails, amputation. "*Wet to dry dressing changes,*" in which a wet gauze is allowed to dry before being removed, is a common technique for removing dead (*necrotic*) and infected tissue. After dead tissue has been removed and the tissue turns bright, beefy red (*granulation tissue*), dressings should be changed to those that remain moist. Many home health agencies supply nurses specialized in treating and healing wounds at home.

A Novel Method of Wound Healing

A recent clinical study conducted in Europe used maggots to clean dead tissue from wounds in people with diabetes, with remarkable success. This technique is not currently being used in the United States, however.

106

Physical Therapy

Physical therapists specialize in the physical retraining of people who have lost function due to paralysis, neurologic illness, immobilization, and prolonged hospitalization. "PT" should be initiated early in the hospital, especially in elderly people or those who have had a stroke, as physical deconditioning can progress rapidly, leaving them unable to return home even when their medical problem has cleared up (many people require a period in a physical rehabilitation center before they can return home). PT is also essential to prevent irreversible contraction of the arms and legs (*contractures*) (also see Chapter 17).

Radiation Therapy

Radiation therapy is used to treat cancer. Large doses of radiation, focused on small areas of the body, can shrink tumors. Radiation therapy is recommended to shrink a tumor before surgery, when a tumor is too large to be removed completely, or when it cannot be removed without damaging surrounding tissues. Radiation therapy doesn't hurt, but it can cause redness, pain, and flaking of the skin (*radiation dermatitis*) and damage to structures around a tumor, including the heart and lungs. Ask your doctor about these side effects—stiffening of the lungs from radiation (*fibrosis*) can cause permanent shortness of breath.

Surgery

Getting your gallbladder out or your nose fixed? See Chapter 12.

Intensive Care

Intensive care, the management of the critically ill, is the subject of Chapter 13.

Following are some good questions and suggestions for your doctor concerning *your treatment*:

Ask the following about IV therapy:

+ Do I really need to receive IV fluid, medicine, or antibiotics, or can I take them by mouth?
+ Do I really need IV nutrition? What happens if I refuse it?
+ Please make sure that my IV is cleaned and changed on a regular basis!
+ I do not want a central line. Is there an alternative, safer type of IV?
+ Do I really need a transfusion, or can I take supplements to build my red blood count? What is my hematocrit? Is it dropping?

The following applies to PEG tubes:
+ Are you certain that I (or my relative) am unable to eat? Please make sure that my (or my relative's) ability to swallow food has been thoroughly assessed before recommending a PEG tube!

The following apply to NG tubes:
+ Will anesthesia be used to numb my nose and throat before the NG tube is put in?
+ Will my NG tube be taken out as soon as it is no longer necessary?
+ Is the suction pump attached to my NG tube set on "intermittent"?
+ Please use a feeding tube, not an NG tube to feed me if I am unable to swallow, and please use it only temporarily!

Ask the following about wound healing:
+ Is my wound clean and is it healing? Please make sure the dressing is being changed as often as necessary!
+ Is it time to switch from wet-to-dry dressing changes to moist dressings?
+ Please arrange for a nurse to visit me at home to help heal my wound.

Chapter 11

Open Wide!
Your Medicine

Doctors can do many things to their hospitalized patients, including operating on them, pumping IV fluids into them, and radiating them, but mostly, they give them medicine. Medicine is dispensed in pill form and through an IV, a catheter in a nose, bladder, or the abdominal wall into the stomach. If you're in the hospital, expect your doctors to give you medicine.

This chapter will introduce you to some of the most common medicines. This is only an overview; only the principle uses and major side effects will be listed. If your doctors want you to use a medication that isn't mentioned here or that you don't know about, *ask* about it. In addition, if you are taking a medication at home, be sure to read the package insert that comes with it or check out the somewhat easier to understand patient information handout that the pharmacy provides.

With Medicine, Less Is Best

Doctors give medicines, and patients expect them. Despite this happy arrangement, remember that less is best when it comes to medicines. Medicines cause all kinds of problems, from allergies and side effects to promoting the development of resistant bacteria; both doctors and patients would do well to exercise a bit of restraint.

When your doctor wants to give you a medication, make sure you really need it. Ask about side effects and toxicities, and if you are taking more than one medication, ask that your doctor check to make sure they are safely used in combination. And if you doctor tells you that you don't need a medicine, be happy that you are being spared the myriad risks medication exposure can create, rather than upset at being denied a perceived, but illusory benefit.

Drug Information at Your Fingertips

ePocrates, a free, downloadable program for handheld computers, lists thousands of drugs, doses, indications, side effects, and has a medication interaction program that will allow you to check that all the medications you are on are safely used in combination. Download it to your Palm or other handheld at www.epocrates.com.

A Medication Primer #1: Routes of Administration

Medication orders are written in shorthand to refer to dose, route of administration, and frequency. Common shorthand notations are shown in the following table.

Medication Order Shorthand

Abbreviation	Meaning
Dose:	
Mcg	Microgram (.000001 gram)
Mg	Milligram (.001 gram)
Ml/cc	Milliliters (.001 liter)
Tsp.	Teaspoon (5 milliliters)
Gm.	Gram

Abbreviation	Meaning
Dose:	
Gr.	Grain (.0648 gram, now rarely used)
Gtt.	Drop
Tab.	Tablet
Cap.	Capsule
† †† †††	One, two, three, and so on
Route:	
IV	Intravenous
PO	Oral
IM	Intramuscular
SQ/SC	Subcutaneous (under the skin)
NC	Nasal cannula
VM	Venti-mask (face mask)
Neb.	Nebulizer
Interval:	
Q1H (Q2H, Q3H, etc.)	Every one hour, every two hours, every three hours, and so on
QD	Once daily
BID	Twice a day
TID	Three times a day
QID	Four times a day
TIW	Three times a week
Qweekly	Once a week

continues

Medication Order Shorthand *continued*

Abbreviation	Meaning
Interval:	
QOD	Every other day
QHS	At bedtime
AC	Before meals
PC	After meals

Routes of administration and preparation of medications include the following:

+ **Oral.** Most medicines are given orally in liquid or tablet form. PO, meaning per oral, is a *very* common medical abbreviation. Tablets come in short and long acting forms; the latter are denoted by initials such as CD, ER, XL, LA, or the abbreviation Contin. (for example, Cardizem CD [diltiazem], Toprol XL [metoprolol], Inderal LA [propanolol], MSContin [morphine], and OxyContin [oxycodone]). Liquid preparations are used for people with difficulty swallowing or those with PEG tubes (see Chapter 9). Many pain and anti-anxiety agents also come in highly concentrated liquid forms that are convenient for people with difficulty swallowing or extreme debilitation from terminal illnesses (for example, Roxanol, containing 100 milligrams of morphine per teaspoon).

+ **Intravenous.** Medications are given IV to achieve rapid, high levels of the medication in the blood, because people are unable to take anything by mouth, or because the medications only come in an IV form. Many of the medications that are routinely given IV *could* be given PO, so make sure to ask your doctor whether the IV route is really necessary. If you *do* need to get the medicine intravenously, ask your doctor or nurse to make sure your IV line is functioning properly before "hanging" the medication, as many medicines, especially potassium, parenteral nutrition, and chemotherapy, can burn or cause damage if they leak into the surrounding tissue (*extravasation*). And make sure to ask your nurse to double-check the dose! A common medical error in hospitals is the accidental administration of IV medicines in much larger doses than intended.

Check Your IV

To see for yourself if your IV line is working, check the clear plastic drip chamber at the bottom of the IV bag. A small steel pin should be dripping fluid into the chamber. The line has a white plastic toggle device to control the rate of drip; when this device is wide open the fluid should drip rapidly into the line. If it doesn't, or if the IV site in your arm is swollen or painful, your IV isn't working properly and should be changed (sometimes, flushing the IV will overcome an obstruction without the need to change it).

+ **Parenteral (through the skin).** Parenteral routes include *subcutaneous* (*sub-Q, SC*), in which medication is injected under the skin but above the muscle, and *intramuscular* (IM), in which the medicine is injected deep into the muscle. Many long acting medications (for example, benzathine penicillin, used to treat a strep throat) are injected "deep IM" where they gradually seep out, maintaining long term, effective levels in the blood stream. Complications of IM and sub-Q injections include pain, cellulitis, and abscess formation.

+ **Epidural and intrathecal.** Epidural medication—injected next to the spine—numbs the lower part of the body and is used to relieve pain during childbirth, caesarian section, and other surgeries. Epidural anesthesia can cause infection and backache, but is generally safe. Intrathecal medication, injected into the fluid bathing the spinal cord, is used to relieve chronic pain, cancer pain, and spasticity from neurologic illness such as multiple sclerosis. Intrathecal infusion pumps are sewn under the skin and left in place for months.

+ **Infusion pumps.** Infusion pumps deliver small amounts of medication over a long period. Cancer chemotherapy and insulin might be given by external infusion pump (carried in a fanny pack); intrathecal pumps are sewn just under the skin.

♦ **Instillation.** Medicines can be *instilled* into body cavities via tubes. People with lung cancer, for example, can accumulate fluid in the chest cavity (*pleural space*) that causes the lungs to collapse. In *pleurodesis,* medication is instilled into the chest cavity to adhere the lining of the lungs to the rib cage and help prevent collapse.

♦ **Rectal.** Suppositories are commonly given to people for the treatment of nausea and vomiting. Suppositories and enemas are also used for the treatment of constipation.

♦ **Topical.** Medications are given topically to deliver antibiotics and anti-inflammatory agents and to assist in wound healing. Topical preparations include the following:

  ♦ **Ointment.** An ointment has an oil base, gives the skin a glistening appearance, and does not easily wash off. Ointments lubricate, soften, and protect skin.

  ♦ **Cream.** Creams are the most common form of topical therapy. They are easily applied and disappear when rubbed into skin.

  ♦ **Lotion.** Lotions are suspensions of powders in water (for example, calamine) or might act like creams. Lotions cool, soothe, and dry skin.

  ♦ **Aerosol.** Aerosols are rarely used to apply medication to skin because creams and lotions work better, although anesthetic spray is useful for numbing mucus membranes such as the nose and throat.

♦ **Nebulizers and Metered Dose Inhalers.** Nebulized medications, used to treat asthma and COPD (chronic obstructive pulmonary disease), are dissolved in water or saline, vaporized with air or oxygen, and inhaled. Inhaled medicines are also given by *metered dose inhaler* (MDI), or "pump." Used properly with an attached *spacer* (Aerochamber), MDIs effectively deliver medication to the lungs.

A Medication Primer #2: Classes of Medicine

Medications can be broadly classified according to category, sub-type, and individual agents. For example: category (antibiotic), sub-type (penicillin), individual agent (amoxicillin).

If you are taking a medication that is not mentioned here, or if you want to know more about a medication, ask your doctor. Another option is to visit the following websites:

+ The Merck Manual at www.merck.com is an excellent source of information about antibiotics, including indications, doses, and side effects.
+ MedlinePlus at www.nlm.nih.gov/medlineplus is also an excellent source of information about medications and all health-related topics.

And remember that when it comes to medications, fewer is better!

Antibiotics

Antibiotics are used to treat bacterial infections. In the past 50 or 60 years, these medications have saved hundreds of millions of lives. Years of indiscriminate antibiotic use, however, have led to the development of antibiotic-resistant bacteria, threatening to throw doctors and patients back to the pre-antibiotic era, in which people with infections either died in a matter of days or weeks or recovered on their own.

In response to this problem, doctors have become more conservative in prescribing antibiotics, and you, as a patient, should participate by avoiding unnecessary antibiotic use. Further, antibiotics can have serious side effects and toxicities; if your doctor is treating you with antibiotics, make sure you *really* need them. If it is possible that you have a viral, rather then a bacterial infection, ask if you might be carefully observed *off* antibiotics, with an eye to starting them immediately if you get worse.

If you are young and free of chronic illnesses that can make you more susceptible to serious infection, this should be a reasonable option. If you *must* be treated with antibiotics, make sure to ask about side effects and toxicities, whether you can be treated with pills rather than with an IV, and tell your doctor you want to be treated for the *least* amount of time possible.

Major antibiotic classes include the following:

+ Penicillins
+ Cephalosporins
+ Aminoglycosides
+ Quinolones
+ Trimethoprim-sulfa (bactrim)
+ Macrolides
+ Tetracyclines
+ Vancomycin

Penicillins

Penicillins are members of the *beta-lactam* family of antibiotics that find many uses both inside and outside the hospital, although bacterial resistance has made penicillins less useful in treating serious infections.

Penicillins are a common cause of allergy and can cause red blood cell breakdown (*hemolytic anemia*) and low white cell and platelet counts. Amoxicillin, ampicillin, and Augmentin are all penicillins; Unasyn is a type of penicillin given IV.

Cephalosporins

Cephalosporins, also members of the beta-lactam family, are the most commonly used class of oral and intravenous antibiotics. Called *broad spectrum* antibiotics because they kill a variety of bacteria, cephalosporins find many in-hospital uses, including the treatment of pneumonia (*ceftriaxone*) and serious infections no longer effectively treated with penicillin.

Cephalosporins have the same side effects as penicillins, and people who are allergic to penicillin have a high rate of cephalosporin allergy. Cephalosporins can also cause severe abdominal cramping and diarrhea (*pseudomembraneous colitis*), especially if used for more than a week. Pseudomembraneous colitis can be caused by *any* antibiotic; as the most commonly used antibiotic, cephaloisporins are the usual culprit.

Aminoglycosides

Aminoglycoside antibiotics can only be given IV and are used to treat *gram-negative* infections (so named because of the appearance of the causative bacteria under the microscope), such as severe pneumonia and surgical wound infections.

Aminoglycosides can damage the kidney and cause renal failure, especially if used for more than a week or in dehydrated patients. *Gentamicin* is a common aminoglycoside; toxicity is reduced by once-a-day dosing and measuring levels of the medication in the blood to assure the dose is not too high.

Quinolones

Quinolones—including ciprofloxacin (Cipro) and levofloxacin (Levoquin)—traditionally used to treat urinary infections, are increasingly being used for other infections. Levofloxacin gets into the blood quickly and effectively when taken by mouth and has few serious side effects (headache, sleep disturbance, and dizziness are the most common).

Trimethoprim-Sulfa (Bactrim)

Bactrim is used in pill and IV form. Once used to treat urinary tract infections, Bactrim is the mainstay of treatment for a common type of pneumonia in AIDS patients (*Pneumocystis carinii pneumonia*, or PCP). Bactrim allergy is very common in people with HIV and also causes anemia and low white blood cell counts (*neutropenia*).

Macrolides

Macrolides include erythromycin, azithromycin (Zithromax), clarithromycin (Biaxin), and clindamycin (Cleocin). Azithromycin is often part of the treatment of pneumonia.

Macolides are notorious for causing upset stomach and diarrhea, and might also cause allergy. Erythromycin is the worst offender, and azithromycin is much easier to tolerate. When given IV, erythromycin can also cause painful inflammation of the vein (*phlebitis*).

Tetracyclines

Like macrolides, tetracyclines can cause stomach upset, diarrhea, and phlebitis, and they *cannot* be used in pregnant women because of the risk of birth defects. Doxycycline (Vibramycin) is used to treat chlamydia, a sexually transmitted infection.

Vancomycin

Vancomycin is one of the biggest guns in your doctor's arsenal and should only be used if you have a severe and immediately life-threatening infection. Vancomycin can cause a severe and irreversible spinning sensation (*vertigo*), especially if used for more than a week. Headache and ringing in the ear (*tinnitus*) are early signs of this side effect; notify your doctor *immediately* if you have either symptom.

Anti-Inflammatory Agents

Anti-inflammatory agents find wide use in the hospital, especially for treatment of autoimmune diseases such as lupus, arthritis, kidney disease, Crohn's disease, and ulcerative colitis, as well as asthma and COPD. Anti-inflammatory agents fall into two categories:

- ♦ Steroids
- ♦ NSAIDS (nonsteroidal anti-inflammatory agents)

Steroids (Corticosteroids)

Corticosteroids are potent anti-inflammatory drugs. Prednisone and Medrol are oral steroids; Solucortef and Solumedrol are IV steroids. IV steroids in large doses are often used to treat asthma;

unfortunately, this practice is not well supported by medical research.

If you are on IV steroids, ask your doctor to make sure that the dose and IV route are truly necessary.

Nonsteroidal Anti-Inflammatory Agents (NSAIDS)

NSAIDs, which combine pain relief, anti-inflammatory effects, and fever reduction, have many good uses, but are also a common cause of stomach ulcers and kidney damage and result in thousands of accidental patient deaths yearly (see Chapter 4). Motrin, Advil (ibuprofen), and Aleve (naproxyn), which are *extremely* common NSAIDs, are available over-the-counter and frequently used in the hospital.

Ask your doctor if what you are getting is a NSAID (ibuprofen is the most common); to prevent toxicity, take as little as possible for only a short a period of time. Do not use NSAIDs if you have stomach or intestinal ulcers, liver disease, a blood clotting abnormality (for example, hemophilia), or alcoholism, and *never* combine two or more NSAIDs (see Chapter 14 for a list of common NSAIDs).

Tylenol

Tylenol works great for pain and fever, but it must be used *only* in recommended doses (see Chapter 4).

Blood Thinners

Blood thinners (*anticoagulants*) are used to treat blood clots in the legs and lungs (*deep venous thrombosis* and *pulmonary embolus*), and to prevent blood clots from forming in patients who are bed bound or have *atrial fibrillation*, an abnormal heart rhythm. Heparin is an injected anticoagulant, and warfarin (Coumadin) is an oral anticoagulant. Your doctor will periodically ask for a blood test to measure your INR (*international normalized ratio*) when you are on coumadin to make sure your blood is neither over- nor underthinned (a usual target INR is 2 to 3).

Low-molecular weight heparin (Fragmin) is a newer and much safer form of heparin that is much less likely to cause bleeding than regular heparin, and does not require repeated blood tests to assure that it is working properly. If you have a blood clot, make sure to ask your doctor about Fragmin.

Cancer Chemotherapy

Most forms of chemotherapy work by interfering with cell division—the process by which tumors grow. Because many normal tissues also regularly divide and replace themselves, this causes many side effects, including anemia, low white blood cell and platelet counts (see Chapter 8), weakness, susceptibility to infection (which can be serious and life threatening), bleeding, nausea, vomiting, diarrhea, stomach upset, hair loss, and oral ulcers.

Susceptibility to infection peaks at one to two weeks after chemotherapy is administered; signs such as fever or cough should be immediately reported to the doctor. Many side effects can be anticipated and treated—especially nausea and vomiting. So if you are on chemotherapy, ask your doctor about side effects and the medications available to help you avoid them.

Erythropoetin (Epogen) is an injected medication that can help prevent chemotherapy-induced anemia, and Neupogen helps prevent low white blood cell counts (see Chapter 15 for more on the treatment of nausea, vomiting, anxiety, and other unpleasant symptoms).

Newer chemotherapeutic agents include *hormone receptor blockers* used for the treatment of breast and prostate cancer, and *immune modifying* drugs such as *interferon*, which alter the function of white blood cells and antibodies. These drugs are less toxic than the older agents, but side effects can be serious. Ask your doctor about their usefulness and toxicities.

Psychiatric Medications (Neuroleptics)

Psychiatric medications are used to treat hallucinations and bizarre thoughts, mania, and depression, as well as to control anxiety, agitation, and delirium associated with medical conditions. Major classes of neuroleptics include phenothiazines (chlorpromazine [Thorazine], fluphenazine [prolixin], and others), and haloperidol (Haldol), as well as newer agents such as risperidone (Risperdal), clozapine (Clozaril), and olanzapine (Zyprexa).

The older agents have a much higher rate of side effects than the newer ones, especially sedation, dry mouth, and disorders of movement. Spasmodic and uncontrollable movement of the mouth, tongue, and lips (tardive dyskinesia) is a side effect that can be permanent. Artane (trihexyphenidyl) and Cogentin (benztropine) are medications given to help prevent these movement disorders. *Neuroleptic malignant syndrome* (NMS), a side effect characterized by confusion, combativeness, fever, and convulsions, can be lethal. Dentrium (dantrolene) is used to counteract NMS.

Make sure to ask about side effects if your doctor recommends a psychiatric medication; if you have a relative or loved one in the hospital who needs sedation, ask the doctor to use an agent with the least likelihood of causing serious side effects, in the lowest possible dose.

Medications Used for Alcohol and Drug Dependence

Alcohol withdrawal syndrome (AWS) is a life-threatening condition. AWS should be treated with *benzodiazepines* (Valium, Librium, and others, see Chapter 15) or *barbiturates (phenobarbital* and others), sedating drugs that will gradually relieve jitteriness and confusion. These drugs should *not* be given on a set dose schedule, as is traditional, but in accordance with the severity of withdrawal based on regular assessment by a doctor.

Neuroleptics, though advised by many for the treatment of AWS, may cause neuroleptic malignant syndrome, which, by mimicking alcohol withdraw may lead the treating physician to erroneously *increase* the neuroleptic dose. Death can result.

Opiate addiction may be treated with methadone in concert with counseling and other treatments aimed at helping the addict get (and stay) clean. Methadone, which lasts 24 hours and does not cause a "high," is given orally and has helped many addicts stop using illicit drugs. Those wishing to stop using methadone may taper gradually off the drug; *clonidine,* an antihypertensive medication, helps reduce withdrawal symptoms such as goose bumps, upset stomach, and difficulty sleeping.

Medications for Pain, Anxiety, Nausea, Diarrhea, and Shortness of Breath

See Chapters 14 and 15 for information on managing these highly unpleasant symptoms.

Anesthetic Agents

You will definitely want to be numb (or asleep) when that appendix finally needs to come out. See Chapter 12 for more information on how.

Following are some good questions and suggestions for your doctor concerning *your medications:*

These apply to *all* medications:

+ Why do I need this medication?
+ What will happen if I don't take this medication?
+ What are this medication's side effects?
+ Can this medication's side effects be treated or prevented?
+ If the side effects are serious, is there a safer alternative medication for me to use?
+ Is this medication safely used in combination with the other medications I am taking?
+ For how long do I have to take this medication?

Ask these questions when medication is administered IV:
+ Must I take this medication through an IV? If possible, I prefer an effective oral form.
+ Please make sure I'm getting the correct dose of this IV medication!
+ Will this medication hurt when I receive it through an IV, and can it damage my vein?

These apply to antibiotics:

♦ Is it *really* necessary for me to take an antibiotic, or am I likely to have a viral, rather than a bacterial, infection?

♦ If it is safe, I prefer to see if I might get better without antibiotics, and to start one immediately if I get worse.

These questions apply to blood thinners:

♦ I prefer to use low-molecular-weight heparin (Fragmin) for my condition, rather than regular heparin.

♦ How often do I have to have my blood checked to make sure the thinning is appropriate?

♦ If I am taking Coumadin (warfarin), what is my INR? Is this too high or too low?

Ask these about chemotherapy:

♦ Does this chemotherapy put me at risk for serious infection? What signs of infection do I need to look out for?

♦ Will this chemotherapy cause nausea and vomiting? If so, please make sure that I am given medications to prevent this side effect!

These questions apply to psychiatric medications:

♦ Can this medication cause tardive dyskinesia or other movement problems?

♦ I prefer to be given a newer psychiatric medication, with the least side effects, in as low a dose as possible.

Chapter 12

You Are Getting Sleepy: The OR and Recovery Room

Surgical practice has changed enormously in the last decade, from the kinds of procedures people undergo to the amount of time they spend in the hospital recuperating. Surgery is one of the most common reasons for hospital admission, so this chapter reviews the basics of surgery. The basics include the measures you can take to avoid complications, ways to recover faster, and how to get home quicker *and* in better condition than when you went in. Isn't that the goal?

Modern Surgery: Smaller, Faster, Safer

The biggest change in modern surgery has been the development of less invasive techniques and reduced in-hospital recovery time. Many surgeries that once required wide incisions and prolonged recuperation are now being performed with fiber-optic devices—long, finger-thick, flexible scopes inserted through inch-long incisions in the abdomen or chest—that allow direct visualization of internal organs. The actual cutting and sewing is accomplished with forceps, also inserted through small incisions adjacent the scope.

Fiber-optic surgeries are shorter and safer, with reduced recuperation time and fewer complications such as blood loss and wound infection. Cholecystectomy (gall bladder removal) is now routinely performed with fiber optics, as is repair of torn cartilage in the knee (*arthroscopy*), exploration of the lining of the lungs (*thoracoscopy*), exploration of the chest (*mediastinoscopy*), and inspection of the abdomen (*laparoscopy*). These operations, which at one time required weeks or even months in the hospital, are now conducted in outpatient centers that send patients home within hours of surgery.

Have such dramatic reductions in hospital stays improved surgical outcomes? *Yes*. The less time you spend in the hospital after surgery the better. By recuperating at home you will be less likely to suffer antibiotic-resistant wound infections, pneumonia, and other complications[1]. But make sure everything you need to recuperate at home is arranged in advance!

You will need an ample supply of gauze, lessons in how to clean and dress your incision, and regular visits from a nurse to assure that you are healing properly. And make sure you have enough medication for pain! Surgeons are notorious for under-treating pain; make it clear in advance that you will not tolerate unnecessary pain.

Surgical Pain

To relieve pain from surgery involving your abdomen or chest, you will need 15 to 60 milligrams of morphine every 2 to 4 hours, or 2 to 10 milligrams of Dilaudid, and somewhere in the neighborhood of half that dose for less invasive procedures. Smaller, older, and more frail people will need lower doses, and younger and more robust patients higher doses. See Chapter 14 for more details.

Surgical Risk

Surgical risk refers to the likelihood that you will develop a complication during or after your operation (the *peri-operative period*). The odds of this happening depends not only on the type and urgency of your surgery, but also on your underlying health. Many complications can develop, but it is the possibility of a heart attack that concerns surgeons the most. This possibility, which is heightened in people with pre-existing heart disease or conditions such as diabetes or high blood pressure that increase the likelihood of heart disease, can even cause worried surgeons to cancel or postpone your planned operation.

Emergency surgery is the riskiest surgery, both because it is often of a type that is dangerous, and because many patients have medical conditions that increase risk, with little time to "tune them up" for an operation (for example, to control blood sugar and blood pressure in people with diabetes and hypertension). Someone undergoing an emergency repair of a ruptured *aortic aneurysm* (dilation and thinning of the main artery in the chest), for example, is not only having his chest opened and losing a pint or more of blood, but he is also likely to be over 60 years of age and suffering from chronic illnesses that increase the risk of heart disease.

Some emergency surgeries, such as appendectomy or drainage of an abscess, are lower risk. Many others, however, are among the riskiest of surgeries, including—to name a few—emergency heart bypass operations, penetrating or blunt trauma of the chest or abdomen with major blood loss (for example, gunshot wounds and car accidents), amputation of gangrenous limbs in diabetics, and surgery in patients who are in shock or have a life-threatening medical problem such as *pulmonary edema* (flooded lungs).

How can you reduce this risk? By its very nature, emergency surgery doesn't give doctors much time to stabilize their patients before sending them to the OR. Beta blocker medicines are given to people with risk factors for heart disease (for example, over the age of 65, diabetes, cigarette smoking, high blood pressure, and others) to help prevent heart attack[2].

Pain control is also *extremely* important. By reducing pulse rate, blood pressure, and anxiety, pain relief significantly reduces post-operative complications including heart attack, blood clots, and poor wound healing[3]. To the extent you are able—the chaotic rush of events that precedes emergency surgery might make communication difficult—make sure to ask your surgeon to aggressively treat your pain in the post-operative period (see Chapter 14). And remember that it is not necessary to withhold pain relief *before* surgery, either. Your surgical condition (for example, appendicitis or cholecystitis) can be accurately diagnosed and treated without forcing you to endure pain before going to the operating room.

Post-Operative Pain

Surgeons combine Demerol and Vistaril on an every-six-hours schedule to treat post-operative pain. Although Demerol does relieve pain, Vistaril will only make you sleepy, and any relief you get from Demerol will last two hours at most, meaning that you will spend four of the six hours in pain. There are many better alternatives, and you should refuse this combination in favor of the medications discussed in Chapter 14.

In contrast to emergency surgery, *elective surgery* is scheduled more in accordance with convenience than necessity. A torn knee ligament might be painful, but it is not life threatening. Most important, it can await the "tuning" of your medical problems so that you are in the best shape possible for the operating room. So reduce *your* risk! Good disease management, prevents all kinds of problems. Now, you have one *more* reason to keep chronic illness under control; maximizing the likelihood that you will recover quickly and uneventfully from an operation.

The Preoperative Period

All surgery, excepting that done as an absolute emergency, will involve preoperative preparation, be it "medical clearance," in which your medical doctor treats any co-existing medical problems to prep you for surgery, or drawing routine bloods and taking a chest x-ray and EKG before elective surgery. You will be forbidden to eat starting at midnight the night before surgery—depending on how busy things are and who's ahead of you in the operating room, this can auger a long and hungry day of waiting—and then wheeled to the waiting area outside the operating room. Fresh in your disposable paper hat (to keep hair from contaminating the operating field) you will be ushered into the OR, asked to shimmy onto the operating table, swabbed with iodine, and your operation will begin.

Eating and Drinking Not Allowed!

Doctors and nurses use the term "NPO" when patients are forbidden to eat or drink.

Types of Surgery

Major surgery is any surgery that involves opening the chest or abdomen. Such surgery takes several hours and will require a month or more for full recovery. Many operations, such as the removal of a tumor of the lung, stomach, or colon, are not amenable to fiber-optic techniques and require wide incisions and many hours in the OR, with prolonged in-hospital recuperation and the risk of wound infections, bed sores, blood clots, pneumonia, and other post-operative complications (see Chapter 17).

A *drain* is a rubber tube your surgeon might leave in the wall of your abdomen or chest to drain blood, bile, or other fluids that would otherwise accumulate after surgery. This tube must be removed before you can go home; another reason your hospital stay might be prolonged. It is even possible that your surgical incision will be left open to allow drainage of infected fluids (for example, when an abscess deep in the abdomen or chest is drained), with a second "stage" operation to close the wound after the infection is controlled.

Chest surgery is even more complicated. Normally, your chest forms an airproof seal that keeps your lungs inflated. When this seal is broken—a gunshot or stab wound will do the job as quickly as an operation—your lungs quickly collapse. A *chest tube* is a rubber hose inserted between your ribs into your chest cavity and attached to a suction apparatus to reinflate your collapsed lungs. After your wounds have resealed, your surgeon can remove the chest tubes without fear that your lungs will again collapse.

Heart surgery is even trickier. Valve replacement and coronary bypass might require that your heart be stopped, and a *heart-lung machine* be used to circulate your blood until the procedure is finished and your heart can be started again. If you have one of your heart valves replaced with an artificial (mechanical) valve, you will have to take a blood thinner (anticoagulant) such as warfarin (Coumadin) to prevent blood clots.

Heart-Lung Machines

Heart surgery and the use of a heart-lung machine can cause persistent memory loss, difficulty concentrating, and difficulty with language comprehension, especially in elderly people[4]. Make sure to ask your cardiac surgeon about these complications and how they might affect you.

Vascular surgery to bypass narrowed or blocked blood vessels and restore blood flow is also a "major" surgery, involving hours in the operating room, extensive blood loss, and wide incisions that are susceptible to infection. Bypass of blocked arteries in the legs is common in people with long-standing or poorly controlled diabetes, conditions that put these patients at even higher risk for problems during or after surgery.

Minor surgery avoids the chest, abdomen, and major blood vessels (although many fiber-optic surgeries in the chest or abdomen might also be considered "minor"), takes less time, involves less blood loss, is less risky, and requires less recuperation than major surgery. Drainage of a superficial abscess and breast enhancement, for example, are significant operations, but they are far less risky than the procedures classified as major surgery, and far more amenable to rapid hospital discharge and home recuperation.

Transfusion

Blood loss is an inherent part of surgery; the bigger the operation, the greater the loss (emergency surgery for trauma or a ruptured aneurysm can involve enormous blood loss). While modern surgical techniques help to minimize blood loss, transfusion may be necessary. Factors that predispose surgeons to transfuse patients during surgery include pre-operative anemia, heart disease (blood loss can reduce oxygen delivery to the heart and increase the risk of heart attack), low blood pressure during surgery, and other factors. Although the risk of being infected with HIV or hepatitis B or C by transfusion is extremely low[5, 6]—and far outweighed by the benefits if blood loss is severe—many people object to transfusion, both for religious and health reasons.

If you are concerned about transfusion, talk with your doctor about the possibility of transfusion-free surgery. Techniques to reduce the likelihood of intra-operative transfusion include building your blood counts before your operation with supplemental iron and folic acid and storing your own blood in the hospital's blood bank for use should you need it during surgery. Trusted friends and family members with your blood type might also donate blood specifically for your use. Blood that is lost during the operation can be collected and recycled with a "cell saver," a device that cleans and reconditions it to be transfused right back into your own body[7].

Anesthesia

Your anesthesiologist is responsible for putting you to sleep (or numbing you up) during surgery and monitoring your overall well-being for the course of your operation. He will watch your blood pressure, pulse, oxygen levels, and heart rhythm, and will be the first to know if you are having a problem.

The type of anesthesia used during your surgery depends on the type of operation you are having, underlying illnesses you might have (such as heart or lung disease), and your own personal preferences. A good anesthesiologist will explain the different possibilities and give you a choice between types. You might also want to take into account your anesthesiologist's own preferences and level of familiarity with a given technique. Although it is assumed by most people (and doctors) that general anesthesia is more dangerous than forms of anesthesia in which patients are not unconscious, or only lightly unconscious (such as regional anesthesia), this has not been proven by research; post-operative pain, nausea, vomiting, and difficulty sleeping, however, have been shown to be more common with general anesthesia[8]. Regional anesthesia might offer the added benefit of up to 24 hours of post-operative pain relief, aiding in pain management in the first day after your operation.

The different types of anesthesia include the following:

- ◆ **General anesthesia.** General anesthesia is used to put people to sleep for the duration of an operation. Most "major" surgeries are customarily performed under general anesthesia. To put you to sleep, the anesthesiologist will give you a cocktail of medications, including a sedative, an opiate, and an agent that will paralyze or render your body completely flaccid during surgery. A respirator will breathe for you while you are paralyzed and unconscious, and you will be kept asleep with a gas such as *halothane*, which is turned off at the end of surgery to allow you to wake up.

- ◆ **Regional anesthesia.** Regional anesthesia numbs up part of your body and does not involve paralysis, being put to sleep (the simultaneous administration of a mild sedative might put you lightly to sleep for the duration of the operation), or the use of a respirator. For people with lung disease such as emphysema, regional might be safer than general anesthesia. In *epidural anesthesia,* medication is injected *next to* the spine rendering everything numb from the mid-chest down. In *spinal anesthesia,* a much smaller amount of medicine is injected *into* the fluid bathing the spine, causing the same effect. But take note! Too much spinal or epidural anesthesia can paralyze the muscles of the chest, make breathing difficult, and result in emergency intubation (placement of a tube in the windpipe) and use of a respirator.

♦ **Anesthesia of a limb.** Limb anesthesia allows surgery to be conducted on an arm or a leg without general or regional anesthesia. In a *nerve block,* local anesthesia is injected into the arm or leg, numbing the nerves that transmit pain to the area requiring surgery.

♦ **Local anesthetics.** Local anesthetics are used to numb individual nerves or a small area of the body. *Lidocaine,* a commonly used local anesthetic, has a numbing effect that lasts for about half an hour to an hour. Local anesthesia is used for dental procedures, small surgeries such as the removal of a small cyst or a skin lesion, and the repair of cuts (*lacerations*) that need stitches in the emergency room.

Prevent Post-Operative Complications

After your operation is over, your anesthesiologist will turn off the gas to wake you up, disconnect the respirator, and pull the tube out of your throat. If you have had epidural or spinal anesthesia, the catheter will be removed from your back (or it might be left in for ongoing pain control). You will then be taken to the recovery room for a period of close observation, or, should you need it, the surgical intensive care unit (SICU). There is no privacy at all in the recovery room, or very little, but this will not matter at all to you as you will still be groggy from anesthesia and remember little of your stay.

Congratulations! You came through with flying colors! But be prepared! Someone just put you to sleep, cut you open, fiddled around with your insides, and then sewed you back together again with bits of nylon. You're going to have at least *some* pain—possibly *lots* of pain—and you're going to thank your lucky stars that you spoke with your surgeon about *aggressive* pain control before you had your operation (remember that pain control is not just a matter of comfort, but also an important element of preventing post-operative complications).

Unless you have had abdominal surgery, you should be able to eat shortly. Post-operative nausea, a potential complication of general anesthesia, can interfere for a day or two but will pass. If you have had an abdominal operation, you will need to start passing gas, and your doctor will need to hear bubbling noises (*bowel sounds*) coming from your intestines before you will be permitted to eat. At first, you will be given broth and other clear fluids, and then you'll advance to regular food. If you are very thin, or if you are unable to eat for more than five to seven days after surgery, you might need parenteral nutrition (see Chapter 10) to maintain your weight and aid in wound healing.

Blood clots are an especially dangerous post-operative problem. Low dose heparin, injected twice daily, helps prevent clots; *alternating compression boots*—inflatable boots which periodically fill with air from a pump and compress the calves—are used in people who cannot receive blood thinners. Getting out of bed prevents both blood clots and bedsores, while an *incentive spirometer* (with its corrugated plastic tube and floating Ping-Pong ball) helps to promote deep inspiration and prevent pneumonia. Make sure to use it several times an hour. And finally, never let anyone touch or dress your surgical wound without *washing his or her hands* first. Insist on this! Better yet, *watch* them wash their hands before they attend you. Hand washing is the single best way to prevent post-operative wound infections, as well as a variety of other infectious complications (see Chapter 17).

Following are some good questions and suggestions for your doctor concerning *surgery:*
+ Please describe my planned operation.
+ How experienced is my surgeon in performing this type of operation, and how often is this operation performed in this hospital?
+ Is my operation high, medium, or low risk for post-operative complications?
+ What are the chances that I will have a heart attack during or after surgery?

+ Do I need a beta blocker medication to reduce my risk of having a heart attack during or after surgery?
+ Am I likely to lose a lot of blood during surgery? Will I need a blood transfusion?
+ Do I need iron or vitamin supplements to build up my blood counts before surgery?
+ Can I store my own blood in the hospital blood bank in case it is needed during surgery?
+ Can my friends or family members donate blood to be used for me if I need it during surgery?
+ Please treat my pain aggressively after surgery, including the use of opiate analgesics in adequate doses. Please do not give me Demerol and Vistaril!
+ Is there a pain specialist available to guide my pain management after surgery, if necessary?
+ Is my blood pressure (or diabetes, or other chronic medical condition) well controlled enough for surgery?
+ Can my post-operative care be conducted at home? If so, please make sure I am provided with the necessary supplies and that a nurse checks in on me to assure I am healing properly.

Following are some good questions and suggestions for your doctor concerning anesthesia:

+ What kind of anesthesia do you recommend for my type of surgery (and medical history)? What are the pros and cons of this type of anesthesia?
+ What alternative types of anesthesia are possible, and what are their pros and cons?
+ What kinds of post-anesthesia side effects can I expect?
+ Can side effects such as nausea and vomiting after anesthesia be prevented with medications? If so, please provide them to me.

These questions apply to the post-operative period:
+ Please provide me with an incentive spirometer after surgery.
+ Please get me out of bed as quickly as possible after surgery.
+ Have you (any doctor, nurse, or other caretaker) washed your hands before examining me or dressing my wound?

Chapter 13

And When You're Really Sick: The Intensive Care and Cardiac Care Units

Most people who are admitted to the hospital have an acute illness (or a flare-up of a chronic illness) that requires a brief period of treatment in a medical or surgical ward followed by discharge home. A minority are *very* sick, and need treatment in a specialized setting such as the *intensive care unit* or *cardiac care unit* (ICU or CCU) that has the equipment and staff necessary to care for the critically ill.

What is critical illness? Critical illness is any medical problem that threatens imminent death. A heart attack that causes massive heart failure (*pump failure* or *cardiogenic shock*), for example, can cause death in a matter of minutes. *Septic shock,* in which overwhelming infection causes blood pressure to collapse, is another imminently life-threatening problem. If patients affected by these conditions are to survive, they need close monitoring, potent intravenous medications, high tech equipment, and skilled personnel to sustain them.

The intensive care unit is a remarkable combination of human skill, space-age technology, and technical know-how that has meaningfully prolonged the lives of many people.

Survival rates for heart attack, shock, multiple trauma, and other high mortality conditions have improved dramatically by virtue of intensive care; and many thousands of people have returned to normal lives because the ICU and CCU were there when they needed them. Unfortunately, these powerful life-sustaining technologies might also needlessly prolong dying, especially among patients who have not provided explicit instructions on the care they wish to receive at the end of life.

An understanding of who will benefit from the ICU/CCU—and who might elect comfort, rather than intensive care—is critical to taking firm control of one's medical destiny. This chapter discusses the nuts and bolts of the ICU/CCU, including practical advice on how to anticipate the outcome of intensive care. (Chapter 19 will examine the issue of when to forgo care, critical and otherwise, in terminal illness)

The ICU and CCU: A Primer

The intensive and cardiac care units are similarly laid out, with one-bedded rooms arranged around a central nurse's station. Privacy is at a minimum, with only a curtain or a large plate glass window separating patients from staff. Each room has a monitor to record blood pressure, pulse, respiratory rate, and oxygen levels, as well as suction and oxygen ports, and other equipment.

What kinds of illnesses are treated in the ICU/CCU? The CCU manages cardiac problems such as heart attack, congestive heart failure, rhythm abnormalities (*arrhythmia*), and pulmonary edema (flooding of the lungs from advanced heart failure); the ICU focuses on critical illness in other organs.

Chest pain is a common reason for admission to the CCU, especially in people with risk factors for heart disease (such as diabetes, high blood pressure, and cigarette smoking) and EKG findings suggestive of heart attack. Even those in whom the diagnosis is not certain might be admitted to the CCU for testing and monitoring, as it is during the first 24 hours that the risk of death from arrhythmia and pump failure is highest.

Ruling *out* heart attack (*rule out myocardial infarction*, R/O MI) with blood tests and continuous monitoring will assure that if the diagnosis *is* heart attack, these complications will be immediately identified and treated. Patients with chest pain but a lesser suspicion for heart disease might be admitted to a *telemetry*, or *step down* unit, where constant heart monitoring is conducted in a less intensive setting.

The ICU sees a broader spectrum of illness and treats a very sick population of patients. People with shock, overdose, sepsis, trauma, or any other life-threatening problem need moment-to-moment, one-on-one treatment not available in the lesser-staffed medical wards. Shortness of breath from asthma, pneumonia, and emphysema are commonly seen in the ICU; lethargy, delirium, and seizures due to meningitis, advanced liver disease, and head trauma are also among the conditions requiring minute-by-minute monitoring and treatment. Overdoses, especially those treated with frequent doses of antidotes (for example, n-acetylcysteine [Mucomyst], given for acetaminophen [Tylenol] overdose) are also best managed in the ICU.

Life Support

When illness worsens *despite* aggressive treatment and close monitoring, life support—the use of machines to maintain vital functions such as respirations and blood pressure—might become necessary. The most common form of life support in the ICU is the respirator (*ventilator*). Most often used when patients are unable to adequately breathe on their own, respirators are also indicated for people at risk for inhaling (*aspirating*) stomach contents and developing pneumonia (for example, a person in a coma after a drug overdose).

Intubation, anchoring a plastic tube (*endotracheal tube*) in the windpipe (*trachea*) to be attached to the respirator, causes gagging and air hunger, and patients who are not tied down or sedated will try to pull the tube out until they become accustomed to the idea of having a machine breathe for them. A minority of patients become dependent on the respirator to breathe. These patients will have a tube inserted into their necks (*tracheostomy*) to be connected directly to the respirator (see Chapter 10).

Patients with very low blood pressure (*shock*) are treated with *dopamine* and *nonepinephrine* (*pressor* medications that stimulate the heart and raise blood pressure), and might have a balloon catheter threaded into the aorta to help the heart "push" blood into the arteries (*intra-aortic balloon pump*). Complications of these therapies are common, especially kidney failure, fluid overload (in which the patient's entire body becomes swollen and boggy, a condition called *anasarca*), and infection. Such therapies cannot be used indefinitely, and patients are gradually "weaned" from them in the hope that they will recover (the doses of medications are reduced and stopped, and the balloon pump is gradually turned off). Patients who are unable to tolerate this process after a few days (that is, to maintain a normal or near normal blood pressure without these potent medications or a balloon pump) are unlikely to leave the ICU alive.

Pacemakers, which can be internal or external, are used to treat very slow pulse rates (*bradycardia*). A temporary pacemaker, literally a pair of electric wires pasted to the skin of the chest and back with large sticky pads, is used on an emergency basis until the more permanent variety—roughly the size of a small beeper—can be implanted under the skin.

ICU Psychosis

ICU psychosis, characterized by agitation, hallucinations, and even violent behavior[1] can result from the loss of privacy and severe illness patients suffer in the ICU/CCU. Modern ICUs, in recognition of this condition, allow curtains to be drawn, lights turned down, and friends and family to visit frequently. Along with treatment of the underlying medical problems that contribute to psychosis, the condition is now less common. (See Chapter 17 for more on hospital and ICU-borne dangers.)

> ### Normal Rhythms of Life
> If you have a loved one in the ICU/CCU, tell the staff you want the normal rhythms of life maintained as much as possible, and that you intend to visit as often as visiting hours allow. Orient your loved one frequently; tell them about the weather, the day's headlines, and bring familiar photos and items from home.

Multi-Organ Failure

Multi-organ failure is the unfortunate ending for many people in the intensive care unit. People with widespread (*metastatic*) cancer, for example, might spend their final days fighting a losing battle against infection, internal bleeding, or other complications of cancer and its treatment. Pneumonia is especially common in this population because of the *immunosuppressive* (immune weakening) effects of chemotherapy. Unlike people with normal immune function, who usually improve rapidly with antibiotics, cancer patients are quickly overwhelmed when bacteria spread through their bodies, causing blood pressure to plummet (*septic shock*). One potent—and toxic—antibiotic is added to the next, and soon patients are tethered to respirators and the many tubes and catheters that supply life-prolonging nutrition and medication.

Disseminated intravascular coagulation (DIC), a blood-clotting problem common in critical illness, leads to bleeding of the gums and blood in the urine, stool, and brain. Toxic medications damage the kidneys (*nephrotoxins*), and patients become swollen and almost unrecognizable. Nurses and doctors, chagrined, but lacking instructions to do otherwise, add drug after drug and machine after machine. When the heart finally stops, chest compressions and electric shock are applied to restart it, but even *cardiopulmonary resuscitation* (CPR) and *advanced cardiac life support* (ACLS) cannot undo extensive damage to multiple organs, and death soon follows.

This scenario is a common one in the ICU. It is the result of good intentions gone wrong, patients who have not fully informed themselves about their condition or made clear to their doctors and loved ones their wishes should they become terminally ill, and doctors who have not asked about their patients' preferences at the end of life[2]. Chapter 19 will discuss how to understand when the battle against illness is lost, and what alternatives there are to the ICU when the diagnosis is terminal.

Cardiopulmonary Resuscitation and Advanced Cardiac Life Support

Death is complete cessation of the heart, a blood pressure of zero, and the absence of respirations. Death can come slowly, as in the previous scenario, or it can come suddenly and without warning, as when an artery in the brain suddenly bursts or a lethal arrhythmia strikes without warning. Whatever the cause, death is permanent if it is allowed to progress for more than a few minutes, leading to irreversible damage to the oxygen-starved brain and heart.

CPR consists of chest compressions and artificial respirations for people whose hearts and lungs have stopped functioning. Advanced Cardiac Life Support adds intubation to the process (placing a tube in the trachea to deliver oxygen directly to the lungs), as well as medications and electric current to restart the heart. *Defibrillation,* in which paddles deliver increasing jolts of electric current to the heart, has been made familiar by television and the movies. Unfortunately, television and the movies have left the impression that "shocking" the heart almost always succeeds, and that a patient, after being successfully "shocked," is out of danger and can resume a normal life.

In reality, CPR and ACLS are most successful in patients who have isolated heart problems. Arrhythmia is the ideal candidate, as the other organs of people affected by arrhythmia are usually healthy, and the heart, after being restarted by medications or electric shock, has a good chance of recovery. Time is of the essence, though, and a delay of even a minute can greatly reduce the chance that a normal heart rhythm will be restored. This is why patients with heart attack are observed in the CCU, where monitors alert staff instantaneously when "sudden death" develops, and ACLS can be started immediately.

Doctor's Code

Doctors refer to death, CPR, and ACLS with the single word "code." "The patient coded" means the patient died, while "we coded him" refers to resuscitating (or attempting to resuscitate) the patient with CPR and ACLS.

Patients with illnesses like widespread cancer and advanced lung disease, on the other hand, respond poorly to CPR and ACLS, even when the heart stoppage is caught quickly. These patients have usually been very sick for long periods and have illness in many organs. Most do respond to CPR and ACLS—that is, a heart rhythm and blood pressure are briefly restored—but the vast majority remain dependant on life support and never regain consciousness. After a period of days to weeks in the ICU, and one infection after the next, they succumb.

Is the ICU for You?

Deciding whether the ICU is for you is a matter of personal preference and what brought you into the hospital to start with. For those who wish to preserve life no matter the chance for long-term survival, the decision is easy; intensive care will be provided regardless of the underlying illness. For those who wish intensive care only if it will restore a level of function that—for them—makes life worthwhile, the decision is trickier, but not as difficult as it might seem. As with all medical decisions, it is based on a trusting relationship with a primary care doctor, a solid understanding of one's medical condition, and a frank discussion of the options.

For people who are free of terminal illness, the decision is straightforward. Critical care is to be provided in all circumstances in which there is a reasonable chance of being restored to normal or near normal function. These "circumstances" are likely to be illnesses that are uncomplicated, limited to one organ system, and easy to treat. An asthmatic, for example, understanding that an attack of wheezing severe enough to warrant the use of a respirator is likely to resolve completely with diligent care and the right medications, elects being put on the respirator if it becomes necessary. Someone with heart disease—knowing that ACLS is likely to restore a normal or near normal heart rhythm—decides to be "shocked" should a heart attack be complicated by arrhythmia.

People with progressive, terminal illness, on the other hand, understanding that recovery is rare in the ICU, might elect thorough and complete, but not intensive care. Someone with advanced cancer, for example, decides to treat pneumonia with antibiotics and oxygen, but not a respirator. Someone with emphysema, understanding the difficulty of getting *off* a respirator and not wishing to be dependent on a machine to stay alive, decides to forgo the respirator in favor of inhaled and intravenous medicines.

Unfortunately, there are no guarantees that these guidelines will work for everyone. Otherwise healthy people with simple pneumonia have died on respirators. People with small heart attacks and arrhythmia have failed to regain consciousness in the CCU after ACLS. Conversely, profoundly ill cancer patients have left the hospital on their own two feet after weeks on a respirator in the ICU and lived many more quality months or years. Each patient is an individual, and no outcome—in the ICU or otherwise—can be predicted with certainty.

Following are some good questions and suggestions for your doctor concerning *intensive care:*

The following apply to patients or their family members/advocates:

♦ Why do I need intensive care? Am I critically ill?

♦ Am I terminally ill?

♦ Am I sick in just one part of my body, or many? Which ones and in what way?

♦ How likely is it that my condition will get better in the ICU?

♦ Am I expected to get worse in the ICU?

♦ Is there a significant chance I will die in the ICU?

♦ What alternatives are there to treating me in the ICU?

♦ Will I need a respirator? If I do, what are the chances that I will later be able to breathe on my own?

♦ Will I need medications or mechanical devices to support my blood pressure? If so, what is the likelihood that my blood pressure will return to normal on its own?

♦ Am I at high risk of developing an infection or some other complication of being in the ICU?

♦ Is it likely that I will need CPR or ACLS?

♦ What are the chances that if I do need CPR or ACLS I will recover?

Chapter 14

Pain Management

Illness causes discomfort in different ways. Nausea, anxiety, shortness of breath, and pain are all symptoms you might encounter during your hospital stay. The prevention and treatment of these symptoms is important not only to your comfort and ability to participate in your care, but also to speed your recovery and get you home sooner. This chapter reviews pain management, emphasizing barriers to effective pain relief and providing easy-to-use pain management fundamentals.

Pain: Undertreated in Hospitals

Pain is notoriously undertreated by doctors and hospitals. Study after study has shown this to be so, including studies of postoperative pain, cancer pain, and just about any other kind of pain you can think of[1]. Why is this so? The biggest reason is the belief that using opiate analgesics for the control of pain leads to drug addiction. Opiates, including morphine, Demerol, Dilaudid, and OxyContin, are *very* effective at relieving pain, especially "big" pain such as that from surgery or cancer. Unfortunately, the widely held, though unfounded, fear of addiction prevents their effective use for the vast majority of patients with pain.

Do opiates lead to addiction? Yes, opiates are *highly* addictive, and every doctor has encountered patients who are addicted to pain medications. Rephrase the question, though, and the answer is very different. Do opiates used appropriately for the relief of pain cause addiction? No! Studies of large numbers of people treated with opiates for both short- and long-term pain have clearly shown that these drugs do not cause addiction when used properly[2].

A *drug addict* is a person whose life revolves around getting and using drugs. Addicts lose their jobs, friends, and families, and, if they do not give up drugs, can lose their lives. Addicts lie, steal, and cheat to get drugs. Most addicts know they are addicted, want to stop, and have tried to stop many times.

People with pain engage in none of these behaviors. Those with acute pain—pain of limited duration—use opiate analgesics until the pain goes away and then go about their lives. If a surgeon allows a patient to self administer morphine through an IV pump after an operation (*patient controlled analgesia,* PCA), for example, the patient uses the drug until the pain is gone and then stops. People with chronic pain use analgesics in a similar fashion to relieve pain and live their lives as best they can.

Patients with pain, especially those with chronic painful conditions such as rheumatoid arthritis or sickle cell anemia, sometimes *seem* like addicts because of the way they are treated by doctors. Doctors undertreat them for pain, so they angrily demand more medication, just like addicts who are trying to get drugs. Doctors give them ineffective nonopiate pain relievers like Tylenol or Motrin, and they *insist* on opiates—just like addicts who are trying to get drugs. People with pain shop around for other doctors, hoping to find one who will finally provide them with relief—just like addicts hunting endlessly for doctors to write them an opiate prescription. When people with pain do use opiates, they sleep a lot and have slowed responses (*psychomotor retardation*), normal and expected opiate side effects, just like drug addicts when they get high.

How can doctors distinguish between these behaviors? Easy. When doctors appropriately prescribe opiates for pain, their patients will eventually reach a dose that provides relief and stop asking for more. Addicts never reach the right "dose," because addiction involves a never-ending upward spiral of drug use.

Patients with pain use their medications responsibly, keep their appointments, and happily cooperate with the pain management suggestions of doctors who are committed to their comfort. Addicts "lose" their prescriptions, demand only one drug (for example, Demerol or Percocet), and show up at the doctor's office unannounced and without an appointment declaring that they need more. (One caveat: People with chronic pain might require escalating doses of opiates after months or years of use. This should not be mistaken for addiction!)

So what's the take-home message? Pain is poorly managed in hospitals—though, to be fair, there *has* been a recent increase in the awareness of the importance of effective pain relief, both in the doctor's office and the hospital. If you are in pain and your doctor suggests that addiction is a concern, be clear about your understanding that this is a misconception and request firmly that your pain be adequately treated. If you have severe pain and your doctor wants to use a nonopiate analgesic, try a dose or two; if it doesn't work, insist that you be given something that *does* work.

Don't argue about which type of opiate pain reliever is used—just about any will relieve your pain if used properly. If your doctor still hesitates (for example, prescribing an opiate dose that is too small or given too infrequently), request a consultation with a pain management specialist who will be better able to assess and appropriately treat your pain. If your doctor is reluctant to involve such a specialist, or if your hospital doesn't have a pain management specialist, get on the phone with patient relations or risk management and complain. The relief of pain in hospitals is a top priority with regulatory authorities such as the state commissioner of health and JCAHO, and any threat to contact them will be taken very seriously.

Another concern doctors have is that opiates cause breathing to slow (*respiratory depression*) and blood pressure to drop to dangerously low levels. As with the concern about addiction, there is some truth in this belief. Opiates *can* cause respiration to slow, and every doctor has treated an addict who overdosed, stopped breathing, and had to be resuscitated. Most have also seen patients who, having erroneously received too *much* opiate for pain relief, also required resuscitation. Once again, though, the *appropriate* use of opiates does not cause this complication, even with the extremely high doses needed to manage very painful conditions. The rule is simple; use enough opiate to relieve pain, and no more. Initial doses should be on the low side, especially in people who are elderly, small, or frail, and higher in those who are healthier and more robust. If this initial dose fails to entirely relieve pain, it should be promptly increased until all pain is gone, and given often enough to prevent pain from recurring. It is the use of *more* medication after the pain is gone—the unnecessary use of medication—that will cause problems such as respiratory depression or addiction.

The bottom line? Expect to be under-treated for pain in the hospital, and insist on effective relief.

Therapeutic Doses

Astonishingly, it is the *non*opiate analgesics that are responsible for most drug-related death in America. Hospitalization and death caused by Tylenol and NSAIDs—used in *therapeutic* doses—far outstrips that due to opiates, a fact that seems to cause most doctors little concern.

How to Choose a Pain Medication: The Analgesic Ladder

Opiates are extremely effective agents for pain, but they are not necessarily your first choice of painkiller. *Which* medication to use is a function of what's causing the pain and how bad it is. A moderate headache, for example, will respond to Tylenol or Motrin, and your doctor's reluctance to prescribe an opiate for this condition is understandable. Post-operative pain, on the other hand, or pain from cancer, requires much more aggressive pain relief, and opiates will be necessary. The World Health Organization's (WHO) "analgesic ladder"[3] recommends mild analgesics for mild pain, working up to the most potent opiates for severe pain.

How to decide which analgesic is right for you? Make it clear to your doctor that you want effective pain relief and that you are well aware of the misconceptions surrounding the use of opiates. Do not insist on an agent, or even a class of drugs, but on *relief,* and work together with your doctor to find the right drug in the right dose.

Pain Medications: A Primer

Pain medications are divided into two classes, nonopiates and opiates. The nonopiates are effective for milder pain, and the opiates for more severe pain. The doses of nonopiates are limited by toxicity, but opiates can be given in as high a dose and as often as necessary to relieve pain—the sky's the limit.

Nonopiates

Used for mild to moderate pain, nonopiates include acetaminophen and the NSAIDs.

Acetaminophen (Tylenol) works for mild to moderate pain and has an additive effect with other pain medicines. Dose is limited because of liver toxicity and should be used with caution in people with hepatitis, cirrhosis, or other types of liver disease. Acetaminophen is often combined with opiate analgesics (such as Percocet or Vicodin) in fixed combinations. Acetaminophen is also contained in many over-the-counter analgesics and pain relievers, making it easy to overdose when combining different agents. Make sure to read the label and never to take two acetaminophen containing preparations at the same time.

NSAIDs (Motrin, Naprosyn, and others) are effective for mild to moderate pain, especially from inflammatory conditions (for example, *rheumatoid arthritis*) and are additive to other pain medications. Many of these medications, including ibuprofen (Motrin, Advil), and naproxyn (Aleve) are also available over-the-counter. NSAIDs can cause life-threatening bleeding in the stomach as well as renal toxicity, especially if used long-term, and should be used with extreme caution in people with bleeding disorders, liver disease, ulcers, and renal disease, or in alcoholics or people who are taking *corticosteroid* medications (for example, Prednisone, see Chapter 11).

If you are concerned about the toxicities of NSAIDS and acetaminophen, ask your doctor whether the pain medication he or she has prescribed is a member of these classes of medications. The Physician's Desk Reference (PDR) provides exhaustive information on every prescription drug on the market (the PDR for nonprescription drugs lists all the over-the-counter medications), including whether the agent that has been prescribed for you is an NSAID or contains acetaminophen (look under "Description" in the drug's entry). You may want to consider making this thousand page tome a part of your library. And make *sure* to take only prescribed doses. It is the commonly held fallacy that over-the-counter medications and pain killers are benign that leads to many a near fatal and fatal overdose.

Opiates

Opiates are used for moderate to severe pain. Dose varies widely, and must be individualized according to response. Patients who have not taken opiates before should start with a small dose (which can be increased until the pain is gone) given often enough so the analgesic effect doesn't wear off before the next dose

Opiates can be given by the intramuscular (IM), intravenous (IV), oral, spinal, and transdermal (through the skin) route. Oral doses must be three to six times higher than IM or IV doses to get the same analgesic effect, while spinal doses (delivered by infusion pump) are much lower. Many of the oral forms come in short and long acting preparations (for example, MSContin [morphine] and OxyContin [oxycodone]) as well as highly concentrated forms for people who have difficulty swallowing (for example, Roxanol [morphine]). The transdermal form, fentanyl (Duragesic) is especially convenient, coming in a patch that is changed every three days. Side effects include nausea, sleepiness, slowed thinking and responses, and constipation. These side effects wear off after seven to ten days, though constipation must be anticipated and treated with stool softeners and laxatives.

There are several different types and preparations of opiates; many of which are described in the following sections. Remember that it is not the dose, or even the agent, that is important when it comes to opiates, but whether your pain is relieved. Expect to be started on a lower dose, to have that dose increased as needed until your pain is relieved, and to be provided the opiate as often as you need it to *stay* out of pain.

PCA (Patient Controlled Analgesia)

PCA is an *excellent* choice for the delivery of opiates to relieve pain, especially severe pain due to cancer or after surgery. In PCA, a pre-filled syringe of morphine (or another opiate) is inserted into an IV pump and *you* press a button to deliver the medication when it is needed. The dose and timing are determined by your doctor (the usual "lockout" is every 15 minutes)—don't let him or her skimp! Patients report much better pain management with PCA versus set dose schedules, and they require less medicine to achieve analgesia[4, 5].

Commonly Used Opiates

Morphine. Morphine is the gold standard by which all other opiates are measured. Morphine may be given IM, IV, or orally, and dose varies enormously. A young, healthy patient who has never used morphine before (*opiate-naive*) might need only 10 milligrams every four hours for complete relief of pain after an appendectomy—and spend the entire day in a deep slumber from the drug's sedating side effect—while a frail elderly person with cancer who has been on the drug for several months might be wide awake and comfortable on a daily dose of 6 grams, 100-fold more than the surgical patient.

Opiate-Induced Constipation

Docusate (Colace), 100 mg three times daily, and senna (Senokot), two tablets daily, along with lots of water, help prevent opiate-induced constipation (see Chapter 15). Drowsiness, although temporary, can be troublesome to people at the end stages of terminal illness. Small doses of amphetamines (for example, methyphenidate [Ritalin]) can be used to reverse this effect (see Chapter 19).

The short acting preparations of morphine (MSIR, Oramorph, Roxanol) must be given every two to four hours to maintain analgesic effect, while the longer acting preparation (MSContin) can be given every 8 to 12 hours. Roxanol, a highly concentrated form of oral morphine (20 mgs of morphine per milliliter in a bottle with a scored dropper), is especially useful for people with difficulty swallowing, and can even be absorbed under the tongue. Like all opiates, morphine causes sedation, slowed thinking and responses, and constipation as side effects, all of which (except constipation, which must be prevented), will wear off in a week to 10 days.

Hydomorphone (Dilaudid) is six to seven times as potent as morphine and may be given by the IM, IV, or oral route. Its high potency makes it especially effective for severe pain from cancer and other chronic, progressive conditions, but it only comes in a short-acting form.

Oxycodone (OxyIR, OxyContin) is equipotent to morphine and is usually administered orally and comes in a short acting (OxyIR) and long acting (OxyContin) form. Percocet combines oxycodone with acetaminophen, limiting the dose to two tablets every four hours; Percodan combines the agent with aspirin, also limiting dose. Oxycodone-only preparations do not have a dose limit.

Fentanyl is a very highly potent opiate that is administered in millionth of a gram doses (micrograms). Used for pain, fentanyl is given as a patch (Duragesic), by an infusion pump that delivers very small doses into the fluid bathing the spine (*intrathecal infusion,* see Chapter 11), or as a lozenge or lollipop (Actiq).

Codeine is rarely used as a stand-alone treatment for pain, although it is effective for cough. When used for pain, codeine is commonly taken in combination with acetaminophen (Tylenol 3 and Tylenol 4), limiting the dose to two tablets every four hours.

Meperidine (Demerol) is usually given IM or IV and provides pain relief for only one to two hours, causing a build-up of toxic metabolites that can lead to anxiety and seizures. The availability of other opiate analgesics makes meperidine a poor choice for pain relief.

Methadone (Dolophine) is a great medication for pain, especially chronic or progressive pain. Methadone's unique effects, not shared by other opiates, result in excellent relief at low doses, even when high doses of other preparations no longer work. Stigmatized by its use for the treatment of addiction, methadone is unfamiliar to most doctors in its role as an analgesic, and you will probably not encounter a doctor other than a pain management specialist who will be willing to prescribe it. Methadone can be very helpful in cancer pain, especially when very high doses of morphine or hydromorphone (Dilaudid) no longer provide adequate relief.

The Sky's the Limit

The sky is truly the limit when using opiates to control pain. Frail, elderly hospice patients with severe cancer pain are not uncommonly treated with over a gram of methadone daily; a dose eight to ten fold higher than that used to treat even hardcore heroin addicts and hundreds of times more than that used to treat lesser degrees of pain.

Other Pain Management Options

Many nonpharmacologic modalities complement the medications used for pain. People with painful physical disabilities from trauma or stroke, for example, benefit from physical therapy to strengthen muscles and restore function. Low back pain also responds to physical therapy, exercise, and weight loss. Psychotherapy, massage, acupuncture, biofeedback, and the judicious use of medications to improve sleep are also helpful adjuncts. Ask your doctor about whether these modalities will help improve your pain.

Surgically cutting nerves or using radio waves to temporarily put them out of action (*nerve ablation*) is performed by anesthesiologists who specialize in pain management. These procedures are only considered in people with severe pain who have not gotten relief with other, less dramatic techniques. Morphine or fentanyl infused directly in the spine by a continuous pump (*intrathecal infusion*) is another procedure performed by anesthesiologists for pain unrelieved by other methods (*intractable pain*).

Neuropathic Pain

Unlike pain caused by damage to tissues that is conveyed by nerves, *neuropathic pain* results from damage to the nerves themselves. Neuropathic pain takes several forms, including "painful numbness," *lancinating* pain (short bursts of intense shooting pain), and *dysesthesia* (pain from normal sensations like light touch).

Neuropathic pain is common in diabetes, alcoholism, and AIDS. Opiates and other traditional pain relievers are less effective at relieving this kind of pain; *tricyclic antidepressants* (for example, *amitriptyline*, Elavil) might help, usually after a few weeks of administration. *Gabapentin* (Neurontin), a newer agent, is also effective, and has few side effects.

Demand Relief!

Whether you are post-op, have cancer, or just have a nasty case of pneumonia, pain will probably be a part of your hospitalization. Despite the increasing recognition among doctors that prompt and effective relief of pain is an important medical priority, there is a good chance that you will be undertreated. Fear of addiction and respiratory depression are common barriers to the effective use of opiates, and many nonopiates are limited by toxicity. Be open with your doctor about your concerns regarding effective pain relief, and be open when it comes to choosing an agent that's right for you.

Following are some good questions and suggestions for your doctor concerning *pain relief*.

These apply to general pain management:

♦ What types of analgesics do you use to treat moderate to severe pain?

♦ I want opiate analgesics if I develop severe pain. Do you have any objection to this? Are you concerned about addiction resulting from pain medications?

Ask the following about nonopiates:

♦ Do I have any conditions that might put me at risk for gastrointestinal bleeding or other toxicities of nonopiate pain relievers?

♦ Please switch me immediately to an opiate analgesic if nonopiates do not relieve my pain, or if there are side effects or toxicities.

Ask the following about opiates:

♦ Are you comfortable and experienced with the use of opiates to relieve pain?

♦ Which opiate will be used to relieve my pain, in what dose, and how often?

♦ Please give me as much opiate analgesia as often as is necessary to relieve my pain. If possible, please put me on patient controlled analgesia for my pain.

♦ Please make sure that I am given medications to prevent constipation from opiates.

Chapter 15

Nausea, Shortness of Breath, and Other Unpleasantries

Pain is not the only nasty symptom you are likely to experience during your hospital stay. Nausea, vomiting, shortness of breath, cough, loss of appetite, constipation, diarrhea, hiccups, itching, depression, and anxiety are all common in hospitalized patients, and, as with pain, they are not always high on the list of your doctor's concerns.

What causes all of this unpleasantness? Sometimes these symptoms are the result of the illness itself. Asthma, for example, directly affects the lung and causes shortness of breath (*dyspnea,* or SOB) as its primary symptom. Likewise, inflammatory bowel disease (see Chapter 9) causes diarrhea, and nausea and vomiting can result from a brain tumor. Just *being* sick causes symptoms, as do many medications. The causes and management of these common symptoms are the subject of this chapter.

Shortness of Breath

Shortness of breath is most often caused by diseases of the heart and lungs such as asthma, emphysema, pneumonia, congestive heart failure, and lung cancer. Treating these illnesses is the best way to relieve this terrible symptom. No matter what the cause, oxygen, when used in the correct amount, also provides relief.

Advanced emphysema, lung cancer, and severe congestive heart failure can cause *permanent* shortness of breath, which might progressively worsen despite the best treatment. People with these illnesses may need long term supplemental oxygen, which can be delivered at home with a *concentrator* that extracts the gas from the air. A back-up oxygen tank is kept on hand in case of an equipment breakdown or power failure.

Home Oxygen Qualifications

Your doctor can determine whether you qualify for home oxygen by measuring an *arterial blood gas* (see Chapter 8). A home health agency will then provide the equipment under his or her direction (see Chapter 1).

Shortness of breath in terminal illness can be relieved with opiates, especially morphine. Morphine, the wonder drug for pain, works like magic for shortness of breath, slowing breathing and pulse, reducing blood pressure, and relieving anxiety. Doses are fairly small, ranging from 2.5 to 20 milligrams every two to four hours.

Nausea and Vomiting

Nausea and vomiting are extremely common in the hospital setting. Conditions that cause nausea and the medications used for relief are described here.

- **General medical illness.** Nausea and vomiting can accompany *any* illness, from heart attack and CHF to pneumonia and AIDS. Treatment includes general measures, such as taking only clear fluids and small amounts of dry food (for example, crackers), and the use of anti-emetic medications such as *prochlorperazine* (Compazine), which can be given by mouth, injection, or suppository. Newer (and more expensive) medications, including Zofran and Kytril, described in the following section, may also be useful.

- **Surgical illness.** Nausea and vomiting accompanied by abdominal pain worse than a routine upset stomach might be a sign of a surgical problem such as blockage of the intestines (*obstruction*) or gallstones. Compazine should provide some relief; even better is the removal of your stomach contents with a nasogastric tube (see Chapter 10). Reglan, which reduces vomiting by causing contractions that help the stomach empty, may *not* be used if there is a suspected blockage because of the risk of rupturing, or *perforating,* your intestines.

- **Gastrointestinal disorders.** Food poisoning, viral irritation of the stomach (*viral gastroenteritis*), medication, and alcohol are common causes of nausea and vomiting (especially when there is no general medical illness to explain the symptom, and stomach pain is only mild). Slowed movement of food from the stomach to the intestines (*gastroparesis*), often caused by ulcer surgery, medicines, and diabetes, might cause chronic nausea and vomiting. Gastroenteritis and food poisoning resolve on their own; *metoclopramide* (Reglan) is used to help the stomach empty in gastroparesis.

Gastric Emptying Study

If you have diabetes and chronic nausea and vomiting, ask your doctor about undergoing a *gastric emptying study*. This test measures the amount of time it takes food to move from the stomach to the intestine. A prolonged gastric emptying time might be the cause of your symptoms, and may respond to medications such as Reglan.

- **Medications.** Medications are a very common cause of nausea or vomiting. *Cancer chemotherapy* is a major culprit; several new and powerful medicines are available to prevent this effect (*dolasetron* [Anzemet], *ondansetron* [Zofran], and *granisetron* [Kytril]) and should be given *before* chemotherapy is administered. Opiates also cause nausea and vomiting, which diminishes by reducing dose or by adding Compazine (opiate-induced nausea wears off after a week or 10 days—see Chapter 14).

* **Cancer, central nervous system disease, and psychiatric illness.** Cancer, diseases of the central nervous system (for example, brain tumors or meningitis), inner ear problems (*labyrinthitis, Meniere's disease*), and psychiatric disorders are among the illnesses likely to cause nausea and vomiting. Nausea associated with cancer might respond to the medications mentioned in the previous paragraph. Tetrahydracannabinol (Marinol), the active ingredient in marijuana, is also used for cancer-associated nausea (and associated loss of appetite). Labyrinthitis and Meniere's disease cause a spinning sensation much like sea sickness (*vertigo*), as well as violent retching; antihistamines (*meclizine* [Antivert], diphenydramine [Benadryl]) and scopolamine (given as a patch, Transderm-Scop), might provide relief.

  Additional agents—usually not associated with the relief of nausea—including haloperidol (Haldol), an anti-psychotic, and *prednisone*, an anti-inflammatory, might also be effective in these and other conditions.

Cough

Cough, like shortness of breath, responds best to the treatment of the underlying cause. Asthma, pneumonia, post-nasal drip, bronchitis, sinusitis, heartburn (acid reflux, or *gastro-esophageal reflux disease*), medications, and cigarette smoking are common causes. ACE inhibitors and beta blockers (including beta blocker eye drops) are medications that commonly cause cough, which will disappear when these medications are discontinued.

Codeine, alone or in combination with guafenesin, may be prescribed to suppress cough (guaifenesin, the active ingredient in Robitussin, is an expectorant, intended to thin and loosen mucus so that it an be coughed up more easily, reducing the frequency of cough).

Loss of Appetite

Decreased food intake for more than a few days causes major
concern for most patients. Although this concern is understandable, most people, especially those who are a normal weight,
can tolerate up to a week with little or no food without any
long-term consequences. If you lose your appetite—a common
response to illness—or if you are forbidden to eat by your doctors, be reassured that you will return to normal eating habits
when you get better.

Water! Water!

People can survive for prolonged periods without food. Being
deprived of water, on the other hand, will result in death in no
more than a few days. Patients who are unable or forbidden
to eat or drink will be provided with intravenous fluid (*saline*,
or salt water) to maintain a normal state of hydration.

Appetite stimulants are available for underweight people
with chronic illness, although the best appetite stimulant is to
restore them as much as possible to good health. People with
AIDS, for example, gain weight as soon as their immune systems start to recover with anti-retroviral medication; people
undergoing cancer treatment usually return to normal or near-
normal eating habits after recovering from surgery or chemotherapy. *Megestrol* (Megace) is used to help put weight on
people with AIDS and Marinol is used to create an appetite in
people on chemotherapy.

Constipation

Constipation might result from medications, especially opiates
and psychotropic agents, prolonged bed rest, dehydration,
reduced intake of food and fluids (and intake of low-fiber
foods), partial blockage of the large intestine, diabetes, a low
functioning thyroid gland (hypothyroidism), multiple sclerosis,
and other illnesses. The best way to treat constipation is to

prevent it by maintaining hydration, getting patients out of bed and on their feet, encouraging a high-fiber diet, and providing bulk laxatives and other medications to promote bowel function (see the following table).

Common Laxatives, Mechanism of Action, and Doses

Category/Name*	Mechanism of Action/Dose
Bulk: Bran powder** Psyllium fiber** (Metamucil)	Increases volume of stool 1 to 2 TB. orally twice a day 3 grams orally twice a day
Osmotic: Lactulose Magnesium citrate Magnesium hydroxide (Milk of Magnesia)	Increase stool water content 1 to 2 TB. orally three times daily initially, then 1 to 2 TB. once a day 8 oz. orally once a day 1 to 2 TB. orally once a day
Surfactant: Docusate (Colace) Mineral oil***	Softens stool 100 mg orally three times daily 1 to 3 TB. orally or rectally once daily
Stimulants: Bisacodyl (Ducolax) Senna Cascara	Cause the large intestine to contract 5 mg orally (10 mg rectally) 1 to 3 times daily 1 to 2 tablets daily 1 tsp. daily

*Laxatives should not be used in patients with intestinal obstruction.

**Take each dose with an 8-oz. glass of water.

***Use mineral oil with caution in the elderly because of the risk of inhalation (aspiration) and lung inflammation.

For those already constipated, a cathartic or stimulant laxative might be needed to make the large intestine forcibly expel stool; if that doesn't work, an enema might be necessary, with manual *disimpaction* as the last resort (i.e., a doctor or nurse dons a latex glove and digs the stool from the affected patient's rectum). Laxatives should *never* be used in suspected cases of intestinal or stomach blockage.

Diarrhea

The majority of cases of diarrhea are viral and get better on their own. Typically, viral diarrhea—known to some as "stomach flu"—is watery, copious, without fever, and might be accompanied by vomiting. When diarrhea is bloody, mucoid, or accompanied by fever, bacterial infection or inflammatory bowel disease (see Chapter 9) should be suspected and will require specific treatment. Serious diarrhea may also be caused by *Clostridium difficile* (c-diff), which is a bacteria that grows in the intestine due to prolonged antibiotic use.

Simple cases of diarrhea resolve on their own; even severe cases will usually require little more than a day or two of IV fluid to prevent dehydration. Anti-diarrheal agents (see the following table) are safely used in mild to moderate cases, but not with bloody stools, fever, evidence of bacterial infection, or signs of serious bowel disease (for example, severe abdominal pain or copious stools).

Table 18.2   Anti-Diarrheal Agents*

Name	Dose
Loperamide (Immodium)	Two 2 mg tablets, then one tablet after each loose stool; maximum of eight tablets daily
Diphenoxylate/atropine (Lomotil)	Two tablets four times daily
Bismuth Subsalicylate (Pepto-Bismol)	Two tablets (two tablespoons) four times daily

Anti-diarrheal agents should not be used when diarrhea is severe or associated with bloody stools, fever, or marked abdominal pain.

Depression and Anxiety

Illness is stressful. Hospitalized people are sick, in pain, away from their normal routines, deprived of privacy, anxious about their recovery, and feeling a loss of control. They might be uncertain about their diagnosis despite test after inconclusive test, expecting the worst. Biopsies take nerve-wracking days to give answers. Unhappiness about this state of events is normal. And given the amount of time spent just sitting around waiting for things to happen in the hospital, there's ample opportunity to think. Anxiety, sadness, fear, and confusion are common among hospitalized patients, who might lose their appetite, have trouble sleeping, and become withdrawn and angry.

Just knowing these feelings are normal can go a long way toward helping you feel better. You are not alone! And, when sympathy is not enough, there's certain to be a psychiatrist in the hospital who'd be happy to provide an understanding ear and a prescription to help you feel a little better. Don't forget to ask if your hospital has patient support groups, especially if you have a chronic or terminal illness. Your hospital also will have a pastor, minister, rabbi, or other individuals to provide spiritual counseling.

The following medications are used for hospital-related stress:

Benzodiazepines (Valium, Librium, Xanax, Ativan) in judicious doses can help relieve anxiety. They are sedating and, like opiates, might cause addiction if used improperly. *Lorazepam* (Ativan) is used for mild anxiety and works for roughly four hours, though this varies widely from person to person. Starting dose is 1 to 2 mgs every 4 hours, or .25 to 1 mg in the elderly (who might have a paradoxical *increase* in anxiety and confusion). *Temazepam* (Restoril) and *zolpidem* (Ambien, a nonbenzodiazepine) are used to help people get to sleep. One note of caution: Benzodiazepines should be used *briefly*. Use for more than a few days can lead to an increase in anxiety between doses, poor sleep, and—eventually—addiction. Anxiety or depression that is persistent should be thoroughly evaluated by a psychiatrist.

Selective serotonin reuptake inhibitors (SSRIs, including *fluoxitine* [Prozac], *paroxitine* [Paxil], *sertraline* [Zoloft]), which might take several weeks to work, are used for more persistent forms of depression and are not appropriate for a brief episode of hospital related anxiety. People with depression related to chronic or terminal diagnoses, however, might benefit from SSRIs, as they have fewer side effects than older agents such as amitriptylene (Elavil) and nortriptylene (Pamelor).

Many medications *cause* depression, including corticosteroids (see Chapter 11), and anti-hypertensive agents. Elderly people on multiple medications are particularly at risk for drug-induced depression. Check the package insert on any medication you are taking to see if depression is a side effect.

Hiccups and Itching

Hiccups (*singulus*), usually brief and benign, can result from a variety of serious illnesses and persist for days or weeks. *Chlorpromazine* (Thorazine) is the drug most commonly used to treat hiccups; cutting the nerve responsible for causing hiccups (*phrenic* nerve) might be a last resort.

> ### Hiccup Cures?
>
> Breath holding, eating sugar, bearing down, gasping (fright stimulus), holding the knees to the chest, and breathing into a bag have all been advocated as cures for hiccups; none have been studied to see if they work.

Itching (pruritis) can be caused by skin conditions including rash due to medication allergy (very common), *contact dermatitis* (for example, a new soap touches the skin and causes a reaction), *cellulitis* (skin infection), and *herpes dermatitis* (herpes rash). Renal failure and blockage of bile flow (for example, from gallstones or a tumor of the bile duct) can also cause itching. *Antihistamines* (for example, *diphenhydramine* [Benadryl], *hydroxyzine* [Atarax]) help itching from allergy; itching from blockage of bile flow might respond to *cholestyramine, rifampicin,* and *naltrexone* (which can interfere with opiate pain relievers), although this type of itching is very difficult to relieve. Many doctors are unfamiliar with the use of these drugs; if you have itching from liver disease or blocked bile flow, make sure to ask your doctor to check into them.

Following are some good questions and suggestions for your doctor concerning *symptom relief:*

- Is my illness likely to cause symptoms such as nausea or shortness of breath? If so, can these symptoms be prevented?
- I am feeling nauseous (short of breath, constipated, depressed, and so on). Is it possible this is resulting from a medication I am taking?
- Are there any medications I am taking or will be taking that are *likely* to cause unpleasant symptoms? What are these symptoms? Can they be prevented?
- Is there a patient support group for my condition?
- Will a psychiatrist be made available if I need one?

These questions relate to cancer chemotherapy:

- What kinds of side effects should I expect from my chemotherapy?
- Does this chemotherapy cause nausea or other side effects? Please make sure that I am pre-treated for them, especially nausea and vomiting!

Chapter 16

It's All Greek to Me: A Primer on Medical Lingo

A lot of what doctors say to each other sounds like Greek, and that's for a reason. It *is* Greek, and Latin, too. *Myocardial infarction,* for example, combines the Greek and Latin words for muscle, heart, and "to stuff" to describe the blockage of blood vessels that causes heart muscle to die—a heart attack.

Effusion, meaning "a collection of fluid," comes from the Latin for "to pour out," and *hemorrhage* comes from the Greek for "blood" and "to break." Of course, the understanding that medical terminology has ancient roots will not help much in terms of deciphering what doctors are saying, unless, unlike most Americans, you happen to be fluent in Latin or Greek. And even being fluent in Greek and Latin won't help you out much with the medical slang and shorthand that floats around hospital hallways.

How, then, to understand your doctor? For starters, don't be cowed by professional jargon. If you do not understand what your doctor is saying, ask him or her to speak in straightforward terms that are easy to understand. The sentence, "A CT-guided needle aspiration of your ovarian mass will be necessary to rule out a malignancy," for example, is unlikely to be fully understood by even the most literate of patients. "You need to have a small specimen taken from the lump on your ovary to make sure you don't have cancer," on the other hand, and, "We'll use a CAT scanner to find the right spot, and then a needle to take the sample," conveys exactly what's going to be done next and why, and there's no reason for you not to insist on the same kind of straightforward language from *your* doctor.

Translators Available

Medical jargon is particularly hard to understand for those patients who don't speak English. But help is on the way! The Patient's Bill of Rights (see Chapter 4) *requires* that the hospital provide translators (including sign language interpreters).

Bringing a paperback medical dictionary to the hospital might further help you understand conversations overheard in the hallway and interpret what is written in your medical record. Online you can check out the www.stedmans.com medical dictionary with definitions of any medical word or term. This chapter will lead you down the right road with an introduction to some basic "medicalese." The chapter will be a short one, though; refer to the glossary for definitions of hundreds of medical words, including frequently used slang.

Medical Stems and Suffixes

Many medical words combine stems that refer to body parts with various suffixes for conditions and procedures. Knowing that *itis* is a suffix for "inflammation," for example, decodes just about every inflammatory condition you might suffer, so long as you also recognize the stem. *Pneumo*nitis? Inflammation of the lung. *Arthr*itis? Inflammation of a joint. *Appendic*itis? Inflammation of the appendix? See?

Common suffixes and examples of their use are included in the following sections.

Conditions

-osis, presence of
  diverticulosis: little pouches on the wall of the large intestine
  endometriosis: uterine tissue outside the uterus
  ecchymosis: a black and blue mark

-itis, inflamed or inflammation
  pneumonitis: inflammation of the lung
  arthritis: inflammation of a joint
  appendicitis: inflammation of the appendix

-lith/lithiasis, stones or calcifications
  nephrolithiasis: kidney stones
  cholelithiasis: gallstones
  phleboliths: calcifications in veins and arteries

Surgical and Other Procedures

-ectomy, removal of
  appendectomy: removal of the appendix
  pneumonectomy: removal of a lung
  lumpectomy: removal of a lump (usually in the breast)
  mastectomy: removal of the breast
  colectomy: removal of the colon (large intestine)
  tonsillectomy: removal of the tonsils

-otomy, a big surgical opening
  laparotomy: opening the abdomen
  thoracotomy: opening the thorax
  craniotomy: opening the skull

-ostomy, a small, semi-permanent or permanent surgically created hole or tract leading through the skin (usually placed to drain a body fluid)
  cystostomy: a hole from the bladder to the skin
  nephrostomy: a hole from the kidney to the skin

colostomy: a hole from the colon to the skin

tracheostomy: a hole from the trachea (windpipe) to the skin.

-centesis, drainage of fluid

paracentesis: removal of fluid from the abdomen

thoracentesis: removal of fluid from the chest cavity

arthrocentesis: removal of fluid from a joint (also known as *joint aspiration*)

-oscopy, use of a fiber-optic scope (see Chapter 12) to explore a body cavity

laparosopy: fiber-optic exploration of the abdomen

thoracoscopy: fiber-optic exploration of the chest (thorax)

arthroscopy: fiber-optic exploration of a joint

colonoscopy: fiber-optic exploration of the colon

esophago-gastro-duodenoscopy (EGD): fiber-optic exploration of the esophagus, stomach, and upper small intestine—a mouthful rendered simple by knowing the rules of the lingo.

Places (Organs and Tissues)

hemo/a-, hemato-, blood

hemothorax: blood in the chest

hematochezia: (also bright red blood per rectum, BRBPR), rectal bleeding

hematemesis: vomiting blood

hematurea: blood in urine

hematoma: a collection of blood

nephro, kidney

nephrotoxic: poisonous to the kidney

pneumo, lung (also "air")

pneumothorax: air trapped between the lining of the lung and the chest wall

pneumonitis: inflammation of the lung

myocardi-, heart

myocarditis: inflammation of the heart

There many others, including *gastro-* (stomach), *duodeno-* (small intestine), *coli/e-* (large intestine, or colon), *ophthal-* (eye), and so on.

So mix 'em and match 'em! Put together the stems and suffixes and come up with dozens more—now self explanatory—medical terms. And don't forget to check the glossary for other common medical words and slang.

Good suggestions for your doctor about medical lingo:

+ Doctor! I don't understand what you are saying about my condition and treatment! Please speak in a way I can understand, so I can choose my care wisely!

Chapter 17

Danger! The Hidden Risks of Your Hospital Stay

Illness is not the only problem you will face while you are hospitalized. The hospital itself poses dangers, which might be far more hazardous to your health. Medical errors, discussed in Chapter 3, are one source of hospital-related (*nosocomial*) danger; bad doctors are another. This chapter describes the most common and threatening of these problems, so you can help your doctors and health-care team avoid making you sicker.

Bad Doctors: Professional Medical Misconduct and Physician Discipline

One of the biggest fears people have on being admitted to the hospital is of encountering an incompetent or unqualified doctor. Poor bedside manners are an annoying reality—and merit a tersely worded letter to the hospital's board of directors—but what you really need to look out for are doctors who have crossed the line with patients (for example, psychiatrists who have had sex with their patients), who are addicted to drugs or alcohol, or who have committed gross errors in practice. There is no perfect way to avoid these behaviors, but you do have some protection. For one, hospital credentialing procedures screen out doctors who have had their licenses suspended or revoked, and continuing medical education requirements help assure that those who are on staff keep up with current medical practice. Furthermore, doctors are required by law to report the misbehavior of other doctors, and they risk losing their own licenses if they don't.

You can also do your own background check on your doctor. A good place to start is your state department of health, which should offer free online access to disciplinary data for all the physicians licensed to practice medicine in your state. Type "physician discipline" in the Search field of your state health department's website, and follow the prompts. Or visit the Federation Physician Data Center, a service of the Federation of State Medical Boards, at www.docinfo.org, for a list of 115,000 actions taken against 35,00 doctors nationwide since 1960. This database covers 800,000 U.S. licensed physicians by name, address, location, and medical specialty. For $9.95 (credit cards accepted online), the Federation will generate a Disciplinary Search Report, listing the type of disciplinary action taken against a physician by state medical boards, the date of the action, the state medical board or licensing agency that initiated the action, and the reason the action was taken. Actions taken by another state or federal regulatory board and sanctions taken by the military are also included.

Hospital Report Cards

In addition to checking your doctor, you might also want to investigate your hospital. The Joint Commission Accrediting Health Care Organizations (JCAHO) evaluates and accredits nearly 19,000 hospitals and health-care programs across the country. An independent, not-for-profit organization, JCAHO is a leader in setting state-of-the art, professionally based standards of practice, and assesses and certifies health care organizations as having met (or missed) these standards. JCAHO's *Directory of Accredited Organizations* is available online at www.jcaho.org/qualitycheck/directry/directry.asp. Access to survey data on your hospital is free, including whether it is fully JCAHO accredited, an overall performance score, individual performance scores across a spectrum of clinical areas, and how it compares with other hospitals. (This search engine is a bit tricky; type the name of your state and city and then choose your hospital from a list.)

A number of other organizations "rate" hospitals, though there is little agreement on how such ratings should be conducted. One hospital might do better than another in measures such as mortality rate and complications, but this might better reflect the underlying patient population than quality of care. With this in mind, check the following list of groups that rate hospitals:

- **Consumer's Checkbook (not-for-profit consumer watchdog group) www.checkbook.org.** *Guide to Hospitals* rates 4,500 hospitals, including mortality rates for ten common conditions compared to national averages. (Cost $19.95, also available online for Consumer's Checkbook magazine subscribers.)
- **Health Grades Inc. (a health-care quality ratings, information, and advisory services company) www.healthgrades. com.** Hospital Report Card rates performance in 25 common procedures and diagnoses for 5,000 hospitals. Also assesses doctors, nursing homes, and home health agencies. (Free online procedure-by-procedure assessment; comprehensive assessment available for $24.95 for three hospitals.)
- *U.S. News & World Report* **(periodical) www.usnews.com.** America's Best Hospitals, ranks 205 hospitals overall, based on mortality, nursing staffing, physician survey, and available services; rates "top" 50 hospitals in 17 practice areas. (Free on the website.)

Common Hospital Dangers and How to Avoid Them

What else can you do to assure your safety in the hospital? The following are among the most common hospital dangers, with practical suggestions on how to reduce your personal exposure.

Hospital-Acquired Infections

Hospital-acquired infections affect millions of people and kill almost 90,000 annually[1,2]. Most susceptible are patients with weakened immune systems and severe illness in the medical and surgical intensive care units. These areas are notorious breeding grounds for virulent bacteria that are resistant to all but the most potent antibiotics. These organisms (including *vancomycin resistant enteroccocus* [VRE], *methcillin resistant staphylococcus aureus* [MRSA] and others) cause wound and urinary tract infections, pneumonia, and sepsis, and can easily lead to death. To prevent hospital-acquired infections for yourself or your loved one, follow these rules.

Insist that everyone who touches or examines you wash his or her hands first. There is no more important advice in this book than the command, "Please wash your hands!" Hand washing is the single most important way to prevent the transmission of infection[3,4]. Routine hand washing with soap and water is the traditional means of disinfection; recent data show that alcohol gels are even more effective at killing microorganisms that cause infection; they are also easier to use and less time-consuming[5,6]. Ask your doctor or nurse to squirt some on his or her hands and wash right in front of you. Whatever you do, make *sure* that everyone who touches you or your loved one washes his or her hands, and that goes *triple* in the ICU/CCU and SICU (surgical intensive care unit).

Refuse unnecessary catheters and tubes. Catheters pose all kinds of risks, especially infection. Bladder catheters (Foley catheters, see Chapter 10), which are commonly placed in elderly patients who are unable to get out of bed to use the toilet, critically ill patients in the ICU, and post-operative patients, pose a serious hazard of bladder and kidney infection. Bladder and kidney infections are the most common type of hospital-acquired infection[7] and they *can* kill! Central lines (see Chapters 1 and 10) can cause collapse of the lung and infection. NG tubes (see Chapter 10) can lead to ulcers of the stomach and esophagus as well as pneumonia.

Although each of these devices has legitimate uses, they *hugely* increase the risk of complications, so make *sure* to ask your doctor whether you (or your loved one) really need them. *Never* let a Foley catheter be placed to assist with hygiene (for example, to prevent you from urinating on yourself or the sheets) for more than a day or two. Patients who are bed bound are far safer if they urinate in a diaper and get cleaned four or five times a day. It is your right to insist on being kept clean—no matter how many times you need to be changed by a nursing attendant—and you should refuse a Foley unless it is absolutely necessary (for example, to measure urine output or to overcome a bladder obstruction).

Condom catheters, which allow for convenient (and sanitary) collection of urine in a bedside bag without the risks of tubes that enter the bladder, are also a good alternative (unfortunately, they only work on men).

Routine central lines, placed in the upper chest (just below the clavicle), neck, or groin (*subclavian, internal jugular,* and *femoral lines*) pose a greater risk of infection than regular IV lines placed in a vein in the arm, while Hickman, Portacath, and PICC lines (see Chapter 1), which are placed under sterile conditions in an operating room, are less dangerous (though usually used only for long term and home therapy). Additionally, Portacaths are buried completely under the skin, making them harder to contaminate than other types of IV lines that extend through and above the skin. The bottom line? Refuse central lines unless they're absolutely necessary!

Remove IV catheters after a maximum of three days. Regular IVs should be left in for a maximum of three days. They should then be removed and a new IV put in at a different site (even if they are working fine, and even if there are no signs of infection, such as redness or pain at the site of insertion). If you *must* have a central line, insist that it be kept clean and dressed and that it be removed as soon as there is any sign of infection (such as redness, tenderness, swelling, or warmth at the site of insertion). Central lines can be left in for longer than regular IVs, but they *must* be kept clean[8]. IV infections are common in hospitals, and it is not unusual for them to lead to serious skin infections and abscesses, amputation of a limb, and even death (especially in people with chronic medical conditions such as diabetes).

Keep IV and wound sites clean. Messy dressings cause infections. Your IV, central line, or surgical wound dressing should be clean and cover the site completely. Dressings that cover sterile wounds (for example, the surgical wound remaining after gall bladder removal) should be changed at least daily. If a dressing comes loose or doesn't cover the wound or site completely, it should be replaced. Nonsterile sites such as infected wounds or drained abscesses should be dressed two or three times daily.

Avoid unnecessary antibiotics. Unnecessary antibiotics kill bacteria that are normal inhabitants of your body and promote the growth of resistant, hospital-acquired bugs that can lead to nasty and difficult to treat infections. If you are on antibiotics, ask your doctor whether you really need them (see Chapter 11).

Bedsores

Bedsores (which many doctors and nurses call "decubitus ulcers") can be disastrous. What started out as a small, nickel sized area of redness at the base of the spine or the hip can turn into a large, ugly, deep wound that is chronically infected and never heals. Elderly people and those suffering from paralysis are most at risk for bedsores, but anyone who is confined to bed for more than a few days, especially people who are comatose and do not move, are at risk.

To prevent bedsores, patients must be turned so no one part of their body is lying on the bed or supporting body weight for more than two hours. The knees must also be prevented from resting against each other (a pillow keeps them nicely separated), and the heels must be *lifted* from the bed. Several different types of mattresses and mattress overlays are available to prevent bedsores, including alternating pressure and air flow mattresses, which reduce the amount of weight supported by any one part of the body[9]. If you or your loved one are immobilized in bed for a prolonged period, make sure to speak to your doctor about having your regular hospital mattress replaced with one of these mattresses.

Blood Clots and Pulmonary Emboli

Blood clots form in the leg veins (*deep venous thrombosis,* DVT) of people who are in bed for more than a day or two (people seated for prolonged periods on bus trips and airplanes are also at risk). In addition to causing pain and swelling, these blood clots can break off and lodge in the lungs, forming life-threatening *pulmonary emboli.* Twice daily heparin injections help prevent clots; people who cannot use heparin (for example, because of the risk of bleeding) wear pneumatic boots that inflate and deflate every few minutes, compressing the veins of the calves. Getting out of bed and walking is another way of avoiding blood clots; people who have been immobilized by a stroke or fracture should be seen by a physical therapist and on their feet as soon as they are able.

Deconditioning and Contractures

Deconditioning is the loss of muscle strength and mass from underuse. *Contractures* are flexed, clawlike arms and legs that result from paralysis and the lack of regular stretching. Elderly people are especially at risk for these problems, especially when confined to bed after a stroke. These patients should be gotten out of bed early and often to prevent deconditioning—an aide or a family member might need to be nearby to prevent falling— and stretching exercises should be instituted immediately after a stroke.

Patients with stroke who have *aphasia* (inability to comprehend spoken words or speak logically) and cannot understand instructions should be provided *passive range of motion* (in other words, regular stretching of the paralyzed limb) to prevent contractures.

The Importance of Advocacy

You were admitted to the hospital to get better, not to go home in worse shape than when you came in. The dangers described in this chapter work *against* this goal; straightforward, consistent advocacy, either for yourself or your loved one, is the best way to avoid them. Refuse unnecessary tubes, IVs, central lines, antibiotics, and procedures! Politely insist that people wash their hands before touching you, and that lines and catheters be removed or replaced! And make *sure* that your elderly relatives are turned in bed to prevent bedsores, provided with heparin or pneumatic compression boots to prevent blood clots, and given physical therapy to prevent deconditioning and contractures! Even better, get them *out* of bed (but don't let them fall!).

In the hospital, as in life, it is the squeaky wheel that gets the grease. Be clear and firm (and polite!) about protecting yourself or your loved one and avoid hospital-borne dangers so you can go home in far better shape than when you went in.

Following are some good questions and suggestions for your doctor concerning *hospital-borne dangers:*

+ Is this IV (central line, Foley catheter, NG tube, and so on) absolutely necessary? If so, when will it be removed? If not, please take it out!
+ Have you washed your hands (doctor, nurse, respiratory tech, and so on)? If not, wash them before touching me!
+ My IV has been in for three days. Change it *today,* please!
+ When will my Foley catheter be removed? Please take it out as soon as it is not necessary! I do not want a Foley catheter for hygiene alone!

These questions apply to stroke, paralysis, or conditions in which you or a loved one might be bed bound:

+ Please make sure that I (or my loved one) am being turned often enough to prevent bedsores! Please make sure that I have an appropriate mattress to further reduce this risk!
+ Please get me (or my loved one) out of bed and into physical therapy ASAP!
+ Please make sure that I (or my loved one) am given heparin to prevent blood clots! If it is unsafe to use heparin in me, please give me pneumatic boots.
+ Please provide me (or my loved one) with stretching exercises to prevent contractures of my paralyzed limb(s).

Chapter 18

Getting on in Years: Hospitalization and the Elderly

Elderly people (those over 65) comprise the single largest group of hospital patients. Elders spend more time in the hospital, are sicker overall, and suffer from more chronic illnesses than their younger counterparts [1, 2]. Although most elderly patients benefit from hospitalization, the dangers discussed in Chapter 17 pose a particular hazard in this age group, and the friend, family member, or loved one of a hospitalized elder must be especially vigilant to help prevent *iatrogenic* (doctor-caused) and *nosocomial* (hospital-caused) injury and death.

The Elderly Patient: Vulnerable to Harm

Why are elderly people at such high risk for harm? Aging causes a progressive decline in the function of each organ system (for example, the heart, lungs, kidneys, eyes, and so on). Even in health, elderly people are functioning near their maximum capacity while going about their day-to-day business. Stress this delicate system, and reserves are quickly depleted.

A healthy young person, for example, can easily tolerate a bad case of pneumonia by using lung reserves to maintain oxygen levels—just as he or she can gulp down enough extra air to chase a bus. Give the same case of pneumonia to a frail elder, and the narrow reserve is soon depleted—just as that elder is unable to sprint after his younger counterpart. Further, many elderly people suffer from chronic illness in several organ systems at once (for example, congestive heart failure and chronic obstructive pulmonary disease), placing additional stress on this highly interdependent system. And not only illness, but the hospital itself adds to the burden already present.

How does the hospital add to the stress of illness? Dangers include[3] the following:

+ **Bed rest.** In the elderly, bed rest leads to rapid muscle deconditioning (10 percent loss of muscle strength per week), decreased blood oxygen levels, loss of bone mass, and contractures. For every day in bed, elders need three days of physical rehabilitation to reverse deconditioning.

+ **Delirium.** Agitation, confusion, disorientation, and even hallucinations occur in 5 to 30 percent of hospitalized elders. Risks factors for delirium include difficulty seeing and hearing, malnutrition, dehydration, unfamiliar surroundings, and the use of multiple medications (*polypharmacy*).

+ **Depression.** Twenty-five percent of hospitalized elderly patients develop depression. Depression can cause memory problems and mood swings suggestive of *dementia* (see Chapter 9), leading to an incorrect diagnosis and the failure of treatment. If your hospitalized elder develops problems (especially memory difficulty) suggestive of dementia, make sure to ask the doctor if depression could be the cause.

+ **Restraints.** Restraints, which might be physical (for example, bed rails and tying the patient down), or chemical (sedation), are used on elderly patients to "protect" them from falls, especially if they are agitated or demented. Unfortunately, restraints *increase* the risk of injury, as well as bedsores and deconditioning, and might worsen delirium.

  Restraints may be *temporarily* necessary in extreme circumstances, such as in an understaffed and busy emergency room, to prevent a fall (and a fracture, worsening immobility) until the elder can be transferred to a better supervised setting.

- **Urinary incontinence.** Urinary incontinence occurs in 40 to 50 percent of previously continent hospitalized elders. The following can cause incontinence: urinary infections, Foley catheters, restraints, bedrails (which prevent the patient from getting out of bed to use the toilet), medications, and alterations in mental functioning.
- **Malnutrition.** Malnutrition is seen in 35 to 65 percent of hospitalized elderly. Causes include changes in diet, dietary restrictions (for example, being prevented from eating before and after surgery), missing dentures, and lack of assistance for people who are unable to feed themselves. Malnutrition contributes to bedsores, poor wound healing, infections, and other complications.
- **Bedsores.** Bedsores of varying degrees are found in 9 to 13 percent of hospitalized elderly patients; 70 percent develop during hospitalization. Bedsores cause a four-fold increase in the risk of dying in the hospital, and increase length of stay. Months of intensive, daily care are necessary to heal bedsores after discharge.
- **Polypharmacy.** Polypharmacy is common in the hospitalized elder, causing allergy (for example, rash, facial swelling, difficulty breathing), side effects (for example, low blood pressure, arrhythmias), and delirium in 10 to 25 percent.

  Elderly people may need a larger number of medications to treat their larger burden of medical problems, but a careful review of most medication regimens by a primary care doctor will usually uncover both redundant and unnecessary mediations prescribed by well meaning specialists.
- **Iatrogenic and nosocomial illness.** Illness caused by doctors' errors and the hospital itself affect 36 to 58 percent of elderly patients. Injuries commonly result from diagnostic and therapeutic procedures (for example, central lines and other invasive procedures), hospital-acquired infections, dehydration, IV fluid overload, abnormalities of blood salt balance (*electrolytes*), and side effects of drugs.

Elderly Dehydration

Elders who have difficulty eating and drinking are especially at risk for dehydration. Symptoms include dryness of the skin, lips, and inside of the mouth (*oral mucosa*), lethargy, and reduced urination. Conversely, those receiving IV fluids and medications are prone to fluid overload, which causes shortness of breath and bubbling respirations (*rales*), boggy skin, and swelling of the ankles and lower legs.

♦ **Falls.** Falls, which can cause fractures, bleeding in the brain (*subdural hematoma*), and other injuries, result from weakness and deconditioning after bed rest, changes in mental functioning, bed rails (for example, when a confused patient attempts to climb over a bed rail and falls), unfamiliar surroundings, flimsy footwear (foam rubber or paper hospital slippers), and lack of walking aids such as canes or walkers.

♦ **Decline in independent function.** Twenty-five percent to 35 percent of hospitalized elders lose the ability to perform one or more *activities of daily living* (ADLs), such as the ability to wash, dress, or use the toilet independently; 15 percent will require nursing home placement.

Avoiding the Dangers of Hospitalization in the Elderly

If you are an elderly person confronting a hospital stay, or if you are the loved one or relative of an elder who might need to be hospitalized, ask the doctor about staying *out* of the hospital if at all possible. Oral medications, close follow-up by phone and in the office, and the use of a home health agency to provide "hospital" care at home are all potential ways to avoid hospitalization.

If you (or your elderly loved one) must be hospitalized, insist on the following precautions:

- **Avoid prolonged bed rest.** Elders should be gotten out of bed early and often to prevent deconditioning, contractures, bedsores, and the many other hazards of bed rest. A physical therapist should be involved within the first few days of hospitalization to help maintain strength and promote physical functioning.
- **Avoid restraints.** Restraints increase, rather than decrease, the likelihood of injury, bedsores, and other problems. Physical restraints should be completely avoided (unless temporary and *absolutely* necessary), and sedation kept to a minimum, with early ambulation encouraged. For those who are unsteady on their feet, a nursing attendant or physical therapist might need to be nearby to prevent falls.
- **Encourage food.** Avoid malnutrition by encouraging and assisting feeding. Dietary restrictions should be kept to a minimum, dentures kept nearby, assistance provided for those who are unable to eat without help, and hospitalization limited to less than two weeks whenever possible. Liquid supplements (for example, Ensure) are of limited benefit and should not replace regular food.
- **Avoid immobilization.** Patients who are unable to move must be repositioned every two hours to avoid bedsores, and weight should not be supported on bony prominences. Stretching paralyzed limbs will help avoid contractures (also see Chapter 17).
- **Avoid falls.** Minimize polypharmacy and the use of sedating drugs and those that cause blood pressure to drop in an upright position (*orthostatic hypotension*), assure grab bars are present in the toilet and shower, and maintain strength, balance, and gait with early physical therapy.
- **Avoid nosocomial and iatrogenic illness and injury.** See Chapter 17 for more information on how to avoid dangers, such as hospital-acquired infections and bleeding from invasive procedures, which are cause by hospitalization itself.

Skilled Nursing Facilities and Long-Term Care

Some elders are unable to return home after hospitalization. An elderly person who lived alone and cared for herself independently and then suffered a disabling stroke, for example, might need a period of physical rehabilitation in a *skilled nursing facility* (SNF) to regain function. If she is still unable to function independently, and if family or friends are unable to make arrangements for care at home, custodial care in a long-term care facility might become necessary (basic needs are met, including bathing, feeding, and using the toilet, but there is no treatment aimed at further recovery).

The Elderly and Nursing Homes

Studies have shown that 43 percent of those who turned age 65 in 1990 will enter a nursing home at some time during their lifetime. Of these, nearly one in three will spend three or more months in a nursing home and one in four will spend one year in a nursing home. It is estimated that one in eleven will spend five years or more in a nursing home[4].

Most health insurance plans and Medicare pay for only limited time in a physical rehabilitation center, with a hefty deductible. Custodial care is not covered at all, and people who do not have *long-term care insurance* (LTCI) have to pay for this service out-of-pocket. Long-term care can be *very* expensive (upwards of $5,000 to $10,000 a month), and those without LCTI will have to "spend down" until they are sufficiently poor to qualify for Medicaid (which *will* pay for long-term care).

Following are some good questions and suggestions for your doctor concerning *hospitalization and the elderly* (also see Chapter 17):

+ Must I (or my elderly relative) be hospitalized? If at all possible, outpatient treatment or home care with close follow-up is preferred.

- Please give me (or my elderly relative) only those medications that are absolutely necessary—the fewer the better.
- Please avoid medications that cause sedation or low blood pressure.
- Please do not use physical restraints or sedation, unless *absolutely* necessary!
- Please allow me (or my elderly relative) to eat an unrestricted and varied diet.
- Please monitor me (or my elderly relative) closely to avoid dehydration or IV fluid overload.
- Please make sure I (or my elderly relative) am seen by a physical therapist and gotten out of bed as soon as (safely) possible.
- Will I (or my elderly relative) need treatment in a skilled nursing facility after hospitalization? Does my insurance cover this expense? What about long-term care?

Medigap Insurance

Medicare pays the full cost of the first 20 days in a skilled nursing facility. A co-pay is required for days 21 through 100 ($101.50 per day in 2002), and longer stays are not covered at all. A Medigap policy can be purchased from a commercial insurance company to cover this deductible. Visit www.medicare.gov and download *Medicare Coverage Of Skilled Nursing Facility Care* for more information (click Index and then click Publications in English). Visit the website of the American Association of Retired Persons at www.aarp.org (click Health and Wellness and then Health Insurance and Medicare) for information on Medigap policies and long-term care insurance.

Chapter 19

When to Say Enough! Terminal Illness, Hospice, and Palliative Care

Doctors are trained to fight illness. And they have done a fine job, bringing about extraordinary advances in diagnosis and treatment in just a few generations. In 1940, for example, pneumonia was incurable. People with the illness were isolated from their neighbors and everyone waited, fingers crossed, to see if they would live or die. Today, the medical armamentarium is mighty, and many once-lethal diseases—including pneumonia—are routinely treated and cured. Significant advances have also been made in the treatment of cancer and advanced heart, lung, and liver disease, meaningfully prolonging the lives of people with these end-stage and terminal afflictions.

Where modern medicine lacks is in the humane and rational management of dying. Doctors, oriented to cure, are ill prepared to deal with the symptoms—both emotional and physical—associated with terminal illness. This chapter reviews the options for end-of-life care, so people with terminal and end-stage afflictions can direct their doctors to focus not only on disease, but also on helping them make the most of the time they have remaining.

Terminal and End-Stage Illness

In general, doctors use the term *end-stage* to refer to the failure of an organ system, and *terminal* when speaking about cancer. End-stage heart failure, for example, describes a decline in heart function so profound that affected patients are exhausted and short of breath after only a minimum of exertion. End-stage liver disease causes fluid accumulation in the abdomen (*ascites*), gastrointestinal bleeding, and other symptoms of liver failure, ultimately resulting in death. Both conditions have very high mortality rates. Fifty percent of patients with end-stage liver disease die within six months[1], and 92 percent of those with end-stage heart failure die within two years[2]. (End-stage renal disease is a notable exception, with people living for years on dialysis.)

Cancer is the condition most people think of when they hear the word *terminal*. Although virtually all malignancies will cause death if untreated, many factors affect survival. Stage, which ranges from 1 to 4 and describes the extent to which a cancer has spread, is the most important. Early-stage cancers are small, confined to one area, and tend to be more curable (this varies for different tumors, though, and some cancers might progress even when caught early); late-stage cancer is more widespread (*metastatic*) and difficult to treat, with stage 4 cancers causing death within months to a year of diagnosis. The underlying health of the affected patient is also critical to treatment and prognosis, because people who are infirm might not be able to withstand the rigors of surgery, chemotherapy, and radiation.

"Cured" of Cancer

When discussing cancer survival, doctors speak of two- and five-year survival rates to describe the percentage of patients who survive for these periods of time. Patients who remain in remission for five years are considered cured from cancer, though "cure" requires less time for some tumors and more for others.

Remember, though, that *survival,* and how *long* someone with a terminal illness might survive, cannot be predicted with certainty. Prognostic estimates are based on large groups of people with a given disease, not individuals. Stage 4 breast cancer, for example, has a very high five-year mortality rate. A doctor who tells a woman with the disease that she will likely die from it will probably be right—unless *that* woman happens to be among the lucky few who survive. Likewise, end-stage congestive heart failure causes the death of most of its victims within a year or two. Some people, though, will defy the odds and live for quite a bit longer. Terminal or no, no one can say for *sure* when death will come.

Accurate Information on Cancer Treatment and Survival

The American Cancer Society has detailed, up-to-date information on the treatment and prognosis of a broad spectrum of cancers at its website, www.cancer.org. Under Patients, Family, & Friends, click treatment options, then Making Treatment Decisions, then Treatment Decision Tools. When you click a specific type of cancer, you are prompted to create an account (at no charge). You will be asked a series of questions about overall health and tumor type (several of these questions are highly medical, and you might have to write them down and get the answers from your doctor).

Once logged in, this site provides you with information on different types of treatment, including basic treatment descriptions, side effects, advantages and disadvantages, as well as whether you (or the person for whom you are researching) are a good candidate for a given treatment. The Treatment Outcomes Tool will bring you through the same series of questions and provide you with specific survival figures—based on up-to-date data from the medical literature—depending on your tumor, overall health, and choice of therapy. If your doctor is not providing you with the information you need, this site is a *very* thorough alternative.

Is *Your* Illness Terminal (or End-Stage)? Ask Your Doctor

How do you know if you have an end-stage or terminal illness? If you have advanced heart, liver, or lung disease such as congestive heart failure, cirrhosis of the liver, or emphysema, and if it has been increasingly interfering with your day-to-day life (for example, causing pain, increasing shortness of breath, or repeated hospital admissions) despite expert consultation and maximum doses of medication, you might have reached the end-stage of the condition. Similarly, if you have cancer that has recurred and progressed despite surgery, chemotherapy, radiation, or a combination of the three—especially if you have been treated several times—the terminal phase has probably begun.

It is time to sit down with your doctor and find out exactly how far the illness has progressed and what average survival rates are for people with your condition. You may even want to have this discussion *before* relapse or progression of your illness. If your doctor hesitates, and if this is information you *really* want to know, make it clear that you want the unalloyed truth, in straightforward terms you can understand.

To get the most accurate information, ask for *average* survival rates—both with and without treatment—rather than how long *you* will survive. Studies have shown that doctors are often overly optimistic when estimating prognosis, especially if they are close to the patient[3]. Asking, "What percentage of people with my illness live for two years?" is more likely to get an accurate answer than "How long will *I* live?" Or ask for a second opinion from a dispassionate doctor who will be better able to objectively assess your medical history and give you truthful information.

Why is it so important to understand prognosis and the likely outcome of treatment? Clear information is essential to making choices about how to spend the time you have remaining. If there is a 70 percent chance of surviving five years with a months long course of treatment that is toxic and painful, for example, most people will probably give it a try. If that chance drops to 5 percent, they might choose therapy oriented to comfort rather than that intended to cure. And even if treatment is not toxic, the meaning of *time,* and how to prioritize work, family, and day-to-day life might change dramatically if the end is in sight. No matter what the choice, you have to *know* to decide what to do.

Active Dying

Doctors are often inaccurate in estimating the long-term prognosis of terminal illnesses. The final 24 to 48 hours of life, however, is a readily recognized period of restlessness, confusion, and "agitated lethargy" known to hospice and palliative care specialists as "active dying."

This book recognizes that different people will choose different types of care at the end of life. Each individual will be influenced by ethical, spiritual, and practical considerations. An emphasis on comfort over cure will not be the first choice for all. Clear prognostic information, however, is important no matter *what* the choice, and this is consistent with the self-advocacy emphasized throughout the book. Some people might want aggressive, life-prolonging therapy no matter what the outcome, others might want no treatment at all; both decisions are formed by an understanding of what to expect as illness progresses. So if you have a life-threatening illness, *ask* your doctor about your prognosis and the likely outcome of treatment, and *use* this information to direct your care.

Having said this, most people will take a shot at being cured when they are first diagnosed with life-threatening illness, and this makes sense. Curable illness should surely be treated, and even if the diagnosis is particularly ominous, conventional therapy is likely to be of at least some help. Aggressive, late-stage cancer might be terminal, but symptoms can be reduced and life prolonged in the majority of cases through the diligent and judicious use of chemotherapy, radiation, and surgery (or some combination of the three), yielding real benefits. Further, the side effects of treatment, such as nausea and pain, can themselves be treated and prevented.

If the cancer progresses and "curative" or "life-prolonging" treatment becomes too physically or emotionally costly or is no longer of help, the focus can shift to more traditional comfort-oriented measures such as analgesics and sedatives. The distinction between "comfort" and "cure," in other words, is not always so distinct, and the two form a continuum, with an early emphasis on prolonging life and a later emphasis on comfort. For those with end-stage disease, the two modalities are one and the same. People with congestive heart failure treat the disease with conventional medications that reduce the work load of the heart and help prevent fluid from building up in the lungs, simultaneously prolonging life and providing comfort by reducing fatigue and shortness of breath.

Advance Directives: The Living Will and Health-Care Proxy

A clear and honest discussion of the options in terminal or end-stage illness, then, is essential to assuring you get the care you want as life comes to a close. *Advance directives,* which direct your doctor if you are in a coma or in some other way unable to advocate for yourself, and which are almost always used by people to refuse life-sustaining therapy at the *very* end of life, are an important part of this equation. Different states have different ways of allowing people to document their wishes during this time, including *living wills* and the *health-care proxy* (or *durable power of attorney for health care*).

Terminally Ill Patients' Rights

The Patient's Self Determination Act, passed by Congress in 1991, established the right of terminally ill patients to refuse medical treatment. This right was codified in the various patient's bill of rights laws passed by the states (see Chapter 5). Though different in their specifics, each bill of rights upholds the patient's ability to direct his or her own care in hospitals and other medical institutions, including care at the end of life.

The Living Will

A *living will* is specific to the end-stage of terminal illness and directs doctors to withhold all care that would serve only to prolong the process of dying, including cardiopulmonary resuscitation and advanced cardiac life support (CPR and ACLS—see Chapter 13), the use of a respirator, artificial nutrition, IV fluids, and antibiotics. Or patients may pick and choose among therapies, electing, for example, to be put on a respirator but not to undergo CPR. Comfort-oriented treatment, such as pain medication, is encouraged in the living will, and patients can change their minds at any time after signing the document. See the following example of a living will from the State of Utah.

Living Will, State of Utah
DIRECTIVE TO PHYSICIANS AND PROVIDERS OF MEDICAL SERVICES
(Pursuant to Section 75-2-1104, UCA)
This directive is made this _____ day of _____, _____.
1. I, _____, being of sound mind, willfully and voluntarily make known my desire that my life not be artificially prolonged by life-sustaining procedures except as I may otherwise provide in this directive.
2. I declare that if at any time I should have an injury, disease, or illness, which is certified in writing to be a terminal condition or persistent vegetative state by two physicians who have personally examined me, and in the opinion of those physicians the application of life-sustaining procedures would serve only to unnaturally prolong the moment of my death and to unnaturally postpone or prolong the dying process, I direct that these procedures be withheld or withdrawn and my death be permitted to occur naturally.
3. I expressly intend this directive to be a final expression of my legal right to refuse medical or surgical treatment and to accept the consequences from this refusal which shall remain in effect notwithstanding my future inability to give current medical directions to treating physicians and other providers of medical services.

continues

---

4. I understand that the term "life-sustaining procedure" includes artificial nutrition and hydration and any other procedures that I specify below to be considered life-sustaining but does not include the administration of medication or the performance of any medical procedure which is intended to provide comfort care or to alleviate pain:

_____

5. I reserve the right to give current medical directions to physicians and other providers of medical services so long as I am able, even though these directions may conflict with the above written directive that life-sustaining procedures be withheld or withdrawn.

6. I understand the full import of this directive and declare that I am emotionally and mentally competent to make this directive.

_____

Declarant's signature

_____

City, County, and State of Residence

We witnesses certify that each of us is 18 years of age or older and each personally witnessed the declarant sign or direct the signing of this directive; that we are acquainted with the declarant and believe him to be of sound mind; that the declarant's desires are as expressed above; that neither of us is a person who signed the above directive on behalf of the declarant; that we are not related to the declarant by blood or marriage nor are we entitled to any portion of declarant's estate according to the laws of intestate succession of this state or under any will or codicil of declarant; that we are not directly financially responsible for declarant's medical care; and that we are not agents of any health care facility in which the declarant may be a patient at the time of signing this directive.

_____

Signature of Witness

_____

Address of Witness

_____

Signature of Witness

_____

Address of Witness

The Health-Care Proxy

A *health-care proxy* is a form appointing an individual (*health-care agent*) to make health-care decisions should a patient become unable to do so him or herself. A health-care agent should be a trusted family member or friend who clearly understands the kinds of decisions the patient would make in a variety of situations. Although the health-care proxy is almost always used in the event of terminal illness, there are other situations in which a health-care agent might be necessary (for example, a car accident that leaves a patient comatose).

As with a living will, the health-care proxy includes specific instructions regarding different therapies, and an alternate agent is listed in case the primary agent is not available. In some states, a health-care proxy is called a *durable power of attorney for health care* or a *medical power of attorney*. The following is an example of a health-care proxy from New York State.

New York State Health-Care Proxy

(1) I,

_____

hereby appoint

_____

(name, home address and telephone number)

_____

as my health care agent to make any and all health care decisions for me, except to the extent that I state otherwise. This proxy shall take effect only when and if I become unable to make my own health care decisions.

(2) Optional: Alternate Agent

If the person I appoint is unable, unwilling or unavailable to act as my health care agent, I hereby appoint

_____

(name, home address and telephone number)

continues

---

as my health care agent to make any and all health care decisions for me, except to the extent that I state otherwise.

(3) Unless I revoke it or state an expiration date or circumstances under which it will expire, this proxy shall remain in effect indefinitely. (*Optional: If you want this proxy to expire, state the date or conditions here.*) This proxy shall expire (*specify date or conditions*):

---

(4) **Optional:** I direct my health care agent to make health care decisions according to my wishes and limitations, as he or she knows or as stated below. (*If you want to limit your agent's authority to make health care decisions for you or to give specific instructions, you may state your wishes or limitations here.*) I direct my health care agent to make health care decisions in accordance with the following limitations and/or instructions (*attach additional pages as necessary*):

In order for your agent to make health care decisions for you about artificial nutrition and hydration (*nourishment and water provided by feeding tube and intravenous line*), your agent must reasonably know your wishes. You can either tell your agent what your wishes are or include them in this section. See instructions for sample language that you could use if you choose to include your wishes on this form, including your wishes about artificial nutrition and hydration.

(5) **Your Identification** (*please print*)

Your Name

Your Signature _____ Date _____

Your Address _____

---

(6) Optional: Organ and/or Tissue Donation
I hereby make an anatomical gift, to be effective upon my death, of: (check any that apply)
❏ Any needed organs and/or tissues
❏ The following organs and/or tissues

_____

_____

❏ Limitations

_____

_____

If you do not state your wishes or instructions about organ and/or tissue donation on this form, it will not be taken to mean that you do not wish to make a donation or prevent a person, who is otherwise authorized by law, to consent to a donation on your behalf.
Your Signature _____ Date _____

(7) Statement by Witnesses (*Witnesses must be 18 years of age or older and cannot be the health care agent or alternate.*)
I declare that the person who signed this document is personally known to me and appears to be of sound mind and acting of his or her own free will. He or she signed (or asked another to sign for him or her) this document in my presence.
Date _____
Name of Witness 1

_____
(print)
Signature _____
Address _____

_____
Date _____
Name of Witness 2

_____
(print)
Signature _____
Address _____

_____

Most states require that advance directives forms be provided to everyone who is admitted to a hospital or nursing home. Instructions for care at the end of life might also be written down, signed, and witnessed, but they should be shown to a doctor (or lawyer) to be sure they are clear and consistent with state laws. Because doctors often ignore people's wishes at the end of life—*despite* their being documented—make it clear to *your* doctor that your advance directives comprise a legal document, and you expect them to be followed.

If your doctor has ethical beliefs that oppose your instructions (for example, he is unwilling to withhold antibiotics or IV fluids), you might need to find someone else to provide your care. Also, make sure the hospital doesn't have any policies contrary to your wishes (as might be the case in hospitals operated by religious orders). If you are admitted to a hospital where the doctors are not familiar to you, make sure to provide them with your advance directives and ask that they be put in your hospital chart.

The not-for-profit Partnership for Caring has free downloads of the advance directives forms of all 50 states—with information on how to complete these forms—at its website, www. partnershipforcaring.org. Click Advance Directives, and then Download State-Specific Documents.

End-of-Life Planning

Last Acts, an organization dedicated to end-of-life issues, on the web at www.lastacts.org, has a thorough discussion of end-of-life planning, including how to discuss end-of-life issues with your doctor, family, and friends, selecting a health-care proxy, therapies to choose (or refuse) at the end of life, life support measures, pain management, and a glossary of terms.

Do-Not-Resuscitate Orders

Do-not-resuscitate (DNR) orders are a type of advance directive that instructs doctors not to perform cardiopulmonary resuscitation (CPR) or advanced cardiac life support (ACLS) if you stop breathing or your heart stops beating. Although a living will or health-care proxy should cover this eventuality, many hospitals and hospice groups request that patients refusing life-sustaining treatment are specific in this regard.

Doctors *will* try to restart your heart and breathing if you have a respiratory or cardiac arrest in the absence of DNR orders (or other forms of advance directives), and signing them will not prevent you from getting lesser forms of treatment, such as antibiotics or IV fluids, that you might still want to have.

Hospice and Palliative Care

Hospice care is designed for terminally ill people who choose comfort-oriented treatment in the last weeks and months of life. Although many people use the word *hospice* to refer to health-care facilities that specifically care for dying people, hospice can also be conducted at home, using a doctor, nurse, social worker, clergy member, bereavement counselor, and even volunteers to provide medical, spiritual, and emotional support to relieve pain, psychic distress, and other symptoms associated with dying.

Hospice uses medications such as analgesics and sedatives for people who have cancer—and *not* chemotherapy—while the spectrum of medications is available for end-stage conditions such as congestive heart failure or cirrhosis of the liver.

Palliative care is more often hospital-based and, ideally, is begun earlier in the course of a terminal illness. Though not specifically oriented to cure, palliative care avails itself of the full spectrum of diagnostic and therapeutic medical modalities (*including* chemotherapy) to maximize the comfort and independence of a terminally ill patient, involve his or her family in care, reduce symptoms such as pain and shortness of breath, prevent rehospitalization, and prolong life without prolonging suffering.

There is a great need for hospice and palliative care in the United States. A study conducted at the Hastings Institute in

1995 found that patients who die in hospitals often experience fear, discomfort, and pain at the end of life. Research has also shown that doctors frequently do not ask about patients' preferences or accurately assess their choices for end-of-life care[4]. Worse, even when people *do* make their wishes clear, they are often ignored[5].

Some people choose to fight terminal illness tooth-and-nail, but, for many, the end of life involves a series of aggressive treatments that were never *chosen* by the patient at all. A diagnosis is made and therapy started, but, as illness progresses, the transition to more comfort-oriented treatment never comes about. Without discussion or choice, the increasingly frail patient is treated and re-treated, complications develop, and he is suddenly in the ICU surrounded by the high-tech gadgetry necessary to sustain life in its most essential form—a pulse, blood pressure, and respiratory rate. Death is inevitable, but it is fought every inch of the way, and every inch is filled with pain and indignity. (The terrifying ICU scenario described in Chapter 13 is an all-too-common one, resulting when doctors and patients fail to communicate on the options for end-of-life care.)

Increased Life Spans

Palliative and hospice care might actually *increase* the life spans of the terminally ill, helping them live *longer* than those treated with potent drugs and respirators in the intensive care setting. Why? By relieving pain, shortness of breath, nausea and vomiting, and other symptoms, stress and the workload of the heart are reduced, *extending* life.

Predictably, many Americans have reacted to the seeming inevitability of the ICU by embracing the "quick exit" of physician-assisted suicide. Hospice and palliative care offers a rational and far more palatable alternative; the promise that dying can be managed and suffering reduced by committed and experienced professionals. This promise is a serious one, and, while total freedom from suffering cannot be guaranteed, sufficient relief can be provided to prevent the vast majority of people from feeling the need to commit suicide.

Terminal sedation, which uses medications (for example, morphine) to render people semi-comatose and pain-free in the last days and hours of life, is an example of the means available to assure this freedom from suffering. Ethically ambiguous on its surface, terminal sedation is *not* intended to take the patient's life—as is assisted suicide or euthanasia (in which the doctor, rather than helping the patient die, actually kills the patient)—but rather to relieve suffering, and its promise should prevent anyone from feeling the need to take his or her own life.

If you are interested in hospice or palliative care, visit the National Hospice and Palliative Care Organization's website at www.nhpco.org to locate a program in your area. Click Find a Hospice Program at their home page and then specify your state and zip code—literally hundreds of programs are listed.

Hospice Insurance

If you want to have hospice care at home, contact your health insurance company to find out what services are covered. If you are a Medicare beneficiary, the Medicare Hospice Benefit will cover a broad range of home-based services, *including* medications for pain control and symptom relief (less a $5 co-pay, in sharp contrast to other forms of Medicare home care, which do not pay for medications at all—see Chapter 1). The Medicare Hospice Benefit, however, will not pay for chemotherapy or for medications for other illnesses (for example, if a Medicare beneficiary has diabetes and breast cancer, morphine for pain from breast cancer is covered, but not chemotherapy to treat the tumor or insulin for diabetes).

The hospice benefit also will pay for a home attendant for four hours a day and a brief period of hospitalization to allow family caretakers—who assume the burden of care—to rest (*respite care*). Download the Medicare Hospice Benefit brochure for more detailed information by visiting www.medicare.gov or calling 1-800-MEDICARE and ask for publication number 02154.

Medicare Hospice Benefit Brochure Online

At www.medicare.gov, click Site Map, scroll down to the Publications section, click Publications in English, then scroll down to Medicare Hospice Benefits and click the View Adobe PDF link. (If you don't have Adobe Acrobat Reader installed on your computer, you can download it for free at www.adobe.com/products/acrobat/readstep.html. When you return to the Medicare website, you will be able to view the 16-page Medicare Hospice Benefits brochure.) This brochure also lists the telephone numbers of all 50 state (and Puerto Rico) hospice organizations.

Insurance coverage for inpatient palliative care is less complicated than that for home-based hospice care, even for Medicare beneficiaries. Managed care companies will want to assure that your hospitalization is medically necessary (see Chapter 3), but, for approved stays, the range of services should be covered, including pain and symptom management, chemotherapy, and medications for other illnesses.

Understanding Denial

The discussion of options for care at the end of life is prefaced on the idea that terminally ill people are ready to confront their illness and make hard decisions about the way they want to spend their remaining months, weeks, or days. Many people, however, will not want to face these issues at all. The word *denial,* much overused in our society, describes the refusal to accept the reality of impending death. Although many people regard denial negatively, it is, for some, the only way to find the necessary equilibrium for day-to-day living and is entirely compatible with compassionate end-of-life care.

Refusing to confront illness merely requires that the choices for care be rephrased. Patients do not *have* to admit they are dying, only to make choices based on a clear explanation of which kinds of treatments are likely to help and which are likely to result in prolonged pain and suffering. To say that chemotherapy will shrink a tumor, prolong life, and reduce pain, for example, is an honest statement, even if the tumor is ultimately incurable. This might sound a bit paternalistic, but it is not. The choice regarding care is still the patient's, put in terms that the patient can understand and consider.

People who care for the terminally ill might find denial to be very frustrating. Bursting with the need to reconcile past wrongs, they are confined by the refusal of their loved one to admit that the time for talking might be limited. "You don't have to say that," is the response to an apology for a long buried slight, "because I'm not going to die."

These feelings of frustration are real. At the same time, terminally ill people *do* know they are seriously ill and possibly dying, even if this is unspoken, and the efforts of the caretakers *are* recognized, even if this, too, is unspoken. So if you have an unresolved issue with a loved one, clear the air before something happens to make reconciliation impossible, whether it is terminal illness, or sudden, unexpected death. If your terminally ill loved one is in denial, tell them you love them, plain and simple. Chances are, they know all is forgiven.

Coma and Vegetative State

Coma is a decrease in level of consciousness so profound that affected patients remain "asleep" no matter how you try to waken them. Neither light, noise, touch, nor pain will elicit a response. Coma follows a severe injury to the brain, be it from head trauma, infections such as meningitis or encephalitis, severe medical illness, deprivation of glucose or oxygen, or tumors. One of the most common causes of coma in the hospital is oxygen deprivation after a cardiac arrest and prolonged cardiopulmonary resuscitation (*anoxic encephalopathy*).

Coma is always a temporary condition, lasting days to weeks, from which patients either recover partially or fully, or go into a *persistent vegetative state* (PVS). In PVS, patients appear to have "woken up" from coma, and will respond to noise and touch, and might even turn toward a voice, but they have no ability to meaningfully interact with others. When they turn toward a voice, it is brief and without any indication that the words have been understood, when they make eye contact, the gaze quickly drifts away without any signs of recognition. Although families often see this "waking up" as a positive sign, patients in vegetative state rarely recover the ability to interact with the world around them.

The odds of recovery from coma are greater in younger people suffering from brief illnesses such as encephalitis or head trauma and lesser in older patients with progressive and irreversible disease such as stroke and Alzheimer's disease. The absence of *brain stem reflexes* (constriction of the pupils to light, centering of the gaze when the head is turned from side-to-side ["doll's eyes"], and blinking when the cornea is touched) is also a poor sign, as is coma that persists for more than four or five days.

Patients who develop prolonged coma and PVS remain bed bound and need around-the-clock care, a PEG tube for feeding (see Chapter 10), and constant attention to prevent bedsores, contractures (see Chapter 17), and blood clots. Pneumonia and urinary infections lead to repeated hospitalizations. Those on respirators might be the subject of emotionally wrenching discussions about ending artificial ventilation and allowing death to ensue.

Brain Death

The term "brain death," although common, is controversial. The absence of *brain stem reflexes* or any spontaneous respirations (very unfavorable prognostic signs) are among the criteria that some doctors use to diagnose this condition.

Like terminal illness, coma and vegetative state present family and friends with difficult decisions regarding care. If you have a loved one in a persistent coma or PVS, talk with your doctor about the odds of recovery. If the withholding of care

such as IV fluids and antibiotics or disconnecting a respirator
are options you wish to consider—after a *thorough* discussion
of the odds of recovery—ask to speak to the hospital's ethics
committee to learn about the options.

Following are some good questions and suggestions for your
doctor concerning *end-of-life care* (also see Chapter 9):

+ Am I terminally ill?
+ Do I have end-stage heart, lung, or liver disease?
+ What are the chances of my surviving two and five years
  with my end-stage disease?
+ What are the chances of my surviving two and five years
  with my cancer, both with and without treatment?
+ If I am not a candidate for curative cancer treatment, will
  palliative chemotherapy, radiation, or surgery help prolong
  my life and reduce my suffering? How much and in what
  way?
+ Am I fit enough to withstand either curative or palliative
  treatment?
+ If I choose to forgo care, will you still be my doctor?
+ Do you have any objections to withholding care such as
  IV fluids and antibiotics, as well as CPR, if I refuse them?
+ Please provide me with living will (or health-care proxy)
  forms.
+ Does the hospital where you admit patients have a palliative care program?
+ Does the hospital where you admit patients allow therapy
  such as IV fluids and antibiotics to be withheld, if that is a
  patient's wishes? Will they allow a respirator to be discon-
  nected?
+ If I choose hospice care at home, can you refer me to a
  local hospice agency? Will you continue to participate in
  my care (for example, by directing nurses who make home
  visits) when I am receiving home hospice care? Will you
  make house calls?
+ Does my insurance cover hospice care?

The following questions are about coma and persistent vegetative state:

- Is my loved one in a coma?
- What is the cause of this coma and what are the odds of recovery?
- Is my loved one in persistent vegetative state? If so, what are the odds of recovery?

Chapter 20

Don't Get Mad, Get Even! How to Complain and How to Sue

People love to threaten to sue other people. Patients in the hospital, stressed by illness and frustrated by sometimes-unresponsive staff and the slow pace of diagnosis and treatment, threaten legal action all the time. Usually the reasons are minor. A doctor is rude or abrupt, a nurse doesn't answer a call bell fast enough, or a diagnostic procedure is cancelled at the last minute. These threats, made in the heat of the moment, amount to little more than the venting of steam in a stressful situation. Still, the influence of lawsuits on the practice of medicine, threatened or otherwise, cannot be underestimated.

Doctors function under a legal cloud. Fearful of missing even the most esoteric of diagnoses or of being held accountable for withholding needed therapy, they push testing and treatment beyond reason, hoping this behavior will protect them from lawsuits (see *defensive medicine* in Chapter 3). Neither practice, unfortunately, will help *you* get better quicker or out of the hospital any faster.

What is the reality of law and medicine? Ultimately, by empowering its readers to effectively advocate for themselves in the medical system and get the best medical care available, this book hopes to *prevent* lawsuits. One way to do this is to practice self-advocacy. Another is to learn how to effectively complain in the hospital, so a gripe never gets a chance to progress to legal action.

But even the best self-advocacy and most effective complaining might not protect you from malpractice, which is why this book will also examine how to recognize when an *annoyance* has crossed the line to a valid reason for a lawsuit.

Listening Is Smart Practice

Doctors who form friendly and collaborative relationships with their patients are not only likely to improve compliance and the outcomes of treatment, but also to reduce the likelihood of being sued—even when they commit malpractice. Patients appreciate being listened to and treated as equals by their doctors, and may show their appreciation by choosing *not* to call a lawyer.

How to Complain in the Hospital

First, to complain effectively, direct your complaint without delay to the person responsible for the problem. If your elderly, bed-bound relative is not being kept clean, speak to the nurse. Be direct, firm, and polite. "I understand that you have several patients to attend and [my relative] might not be your first priority. Still, he/she is unable to clean him/herself and it has been two hours since the sheets were changed. Please make sure he/she is cleaned up immediately."

A firm, yet polite tone will engage staff in a positive manner and avoid resentment. Hospital workers, especially nursing and clerical staff, are largely unrecognized for their hard work and long hours, and they will be grateful for your respectful tone. Yelling angrily will also get results, but, as mentioned in Chapter 7, it might also cause staff to keep their distance.

If this doesn't get you the response you need, bring your complaint to a supervisor. If the nurse has not responded to your plea within 15 minutes, speak to the head nurse or nursing supervisor (often referred to as the *nursing care coordinator,* or NCC). Once again, make your complaint firm and clear, and insist that it be attended promptly.

If you have brought your complaint to supervisory staff without satisfaction, or if you have complained without avail to your attending doctor, it is time to appeal at a higher level. The patient representative is specifically enjoined to respond to complaints, but does not have the heft of senior administrative staff. Call them first, and then move right on to risk management (the hospital lawyers), the head of nursing, the chief operating officer, the chief executive officer, and even the head of the board of trustees (telephone numbers should be available through the hospital operator).

Make it clear that you expect your problem to be fixed *today* or you will go to outside authorities. Cold food is not a reason to make this threat, but unsanitary conditions or anything else that threatens your safety or that of your loved one (see Chapters 17 and 18) *is*. Senior hospital personnel take patient complaints *very* seriously and have the authority to make people move very quickly to fix the problem. They will respond immediately to the threat to bring in outside authorities, and your problem will be solved.

Complaining to Outside Authorities

If you choose to complain to "outside authorities," the Joint Commission Accrediting Healthcare Organizations (JCAHO) is the place to go. JCAHO is *the* heavy hitter in hospital standard setting and accreditation. If you complaint to them, the hospital *must* respond, demonstrating not only that it has addressed your problem, but also that the same kind of problem will not happen to others in the future (for example, if your elderly relative wasn't kept clean, the hospital might have to prioritize patient cleanliness and send JCAHO a plan of action in this regard). To complain to JCAHO, e-mail complaint@jcaho.org.

To complain about a doctor (rather than the institution as a whole), you will need to identify the agency that handles professional discipline in your state. Complaints are usually handled by the department of health or education, the state medical board, or the state board of medical examiners. The health department or state medical board website will have more information or an e-mail address and telephone number for inquiries.

Although complaining to outside authorities is certain to get the hospital administration to sit up and listen, it is unlikely to get the quick action necessary to fix the problem at the moment. Outside regulatory authorities might take a month or more to respond to your complaint, by which time you (or your loved one) will have long since been discharged from the hospital. So if at all possible, try to resolve your complaint by dealing directly with hospital personnel.

When to Sue Your Doctor

When shouldn't you escalate from complaining to suing? Good reasons *not* to sue include the following:
  + Your doctor was rude.
  + Your nurse was rude.
  + The guy from the transportation department who wheeled you down to x-ray was rude.
  + Your food was cold/moldy/bad/absent.
  + No one would answer your questions.
  + You got tired of sitting in the waiting area outside the emergency room and stormed out in a huff.
  + You had a bad outcome (including *death*) despite receiving the best care.

Here are some reasons *to* sue:
  + You had chest pain, they didn't do an EKG, and you had a disabling heart attack.
  + They misdiagnosed appendicitis as an upset stomach and two weeks later operated on you for an abscess the size of a cantaloupe.
  + Your doctor misread your chest x-ray and two years later you found out it showed a cancer that is now inoperable.

Rudeness merits a tersely worded letter of complaint. Incompetence, unnecessary suffering, and death resulting from negligence or error merit a lawsuit.

Suing is not merely a matter of walking into a lawyer's office and demanding a lawsuit be filed. The administrative costs of litigation can run into tens of thousands of dollars (or more), and your lawyer is going to want some assurance that these costs, and more, are going to be recouped.

A Mistake Must Have Been Made

For your lawsuit to be successful, you must prove that your doctor made a mistake in your care. Usually, this means that another doctor (an *expert witness*) will be hired to review your medical records and give an opinion on the care you received. If the expert agrees that your doctor erred, your lawyer will claim there has been a "breach in the standard of practice" and that a "reasonable and prudent" physician would have conducted your care differently.

What is important is not the *outcome* (presumably, though, the outcome was bad, otherwise you wouldn't be suing), but that a mistake was made. As an example, say you had a serious and painful wound infection after a routine operation that prolonged your hospitalization and interfered with your ability to return to work. If the surgery was conducted properly and your surgeon did everything possible to prevent you from getting an infection and then treated it properly once it developed, and if you signed a consent form indicating you knew an infection might occur, you will have trouble proving malpractice occurred.

If, on the other hand, you received poor post-operative care and your surgeon failed to respond properly to a developing infection, you will have a good lawsuit whether you were warned about the possibility of an infection or not. (This is why you don't have to worry about your ability to sue after signing an informed consent form. Informed consent, done properly (see Chapter 5) means that you are aware a bad outcome is possible, not that your doctor is free to make mistakes or practice bad medicine.)

It is very important to emphasize that a bad outcome, such as death or suffering, is not in and of itself a reason to sue. Doctors are not miracle workers. Bad outcomes, including death, can happen despite the best medical practice. Rather, a doctor must have practiced bad medicine—medicine that would *not* have been performed by a reasonable and prudent physician—and *that* is why the bad outcome came about.

It is also true that a bad outcome *can* be a reason to sue, even if good medicine was practiced, if you were not fully informed about all the possibilities. Surgery, for example, can be complicated and messy. People can have lethal reactions to anesthesia, unforeseen complications can arise in the operating room (for example, a simple fiber-optic [*laparoscopic*] gall bladder removal [*cholecystectomy*] causes bleeding that necessitates a wide incision and prolonged post-operative recovery), wounds can become infected, and so on. If you were not informed of these possibilities—and given the chance to decide *not* to undergo surgery and *avoid* potential complications—you may have a good reason to sue. This is one reason that *truly* informed consent (Chapter 5) is so important.

Mistakes come in several forms, including the following:

- ◆ Failure to properly diagnose and treat a condition (for example, you had chest pain, your doctor sent you home without doing an EKG, and you later went to the emergency room with a heart attack).
- ◆ Obvious mistakes in treatment (for example, your surgeon accidentally severed a nerve, causing loss of sensation or paralysis).
- ◆ A serious condition was not followed-up (for example, you had a small mass on your chest x-ray but were not told that this needed follow-up, later, you were diagnosed with a large, inoperable lung tumor).
- ◆ Informed consent was not conducted properly (see example before this list).

There Must Have Been an Injury Resulting from This Mistake

Even if a mistake was made, you will have trouble winning damages if it can't be proved that this led to an injury. If your doctor failed to tell you about a mass on your chest x-ray, that error is not significant if the tumor was already inoperable when the x-ray was taken. Or say the tumor *is* operable (*despite* a delay in diagnosis), and the cancer is removed and you are cured. Other than a brief period of anxiety over a missed opportunity for earlier treatment, there is no *injury*, and little basis for a lawsuit.

There Must Be Damages Resulting from the Mistake

Not only must you show that there has been a mistake and an injury, but also that monetary compensation is an appropriate response. If your surgical wound infection led to prolonged pain and a delay in your returning to work, as well a stack of extra medical bills, you should be entitled to compensation for your lost income, pain and suffering, and extra expenses. If the failure to follow-up on the mass on your chest x-ray led to your premature death, your survivors might be entitled a payment equal to the money you *would* have earned had you lived.

Lost income and pain and suffering are the main considerations a jury takes into account when assessing damages. As cruel as it might sound, a mistake leading to the sudden and painless death of an individual with no income (for example, a mentally retarded person) might lead to little or no compensation, because there was no lost income and no pain and suffering.

What to Expect If You Do Sue

If you do have a valid claim of medical malpractice, bear in mind that there is a statute of limitations on claims, and an attorney should file your suit within two years of the occurrence. You will have to undergo a *deposition*, in which your doctor's lawyer will ask you questions under oath to try and poke holes in your case. Also, it might take *years* for your case to wend its way through the legal system (three to five years would not be unusual).

If you have a good case, the insurance company representing your doctor will probably offer to settle your claim out of court rather than risk a large jury award. If your case is *really* good, you might want to go to trial anyway, on the presumption that the jury will find in your favor and award you more money. But be warned! More than 70 percent of malpractice cases that do go to trial are found to be without merit and thrown out by the judge or jury. And if the jury *doesn't* find in your favor, you get nothing, not even the settlement offer.

Should you sue? *HealthSmart Hospital Handbook* recognizes and supports the right of people to sue their doctors if an error has been made, an injury has resulted, and there are valid damages. *HealthSmart Hospital Handbook* also recognizes that ever increasing malpractice premiums, spurious lawsuits, and unreasonable jury awards—which can reach millions of dollars for pain and suffering—are a real problem, driving doctors from providing high-risk care, increasing medical costs, and burdening the legal system.

Hopefully, readers will avoid the situations that lead to lawsuits. But if a serious mistake has been made, the information in this chapter should be of help in knowing when a lawsuit is appropriate.

Following are some good questions and suggestions for your doctor concerning *complaints and lawsuits:*

- ♦ Can you provide me with a telephone number where I can reach you, or leave a message for you, in case I have a question or a problem during my treatment in the hospital?
- ♦ Have you ever been sued for malpractice? If so, why? What was the outcome of the suit? Do you feel you were sued unfairly, and, if so, why?
- ♦ Please do not practice "defensive medicine" in my care! I am interested in being informed about my condition and in making good choices about my care, not in being "litigious" or filing frivolous lawsuits.
- ♦ Please *fully* inform me of the potential complications of my treatment, as well as the alternatives to treatment, so I can decide whether the benefits of my treatment outweigh the possible risks.

Chapter 21

Parting Is Such Sweet Sorrow: Hospital Discharge

You made it! You had a problem, got admitted, got better, and now it's time to go home. What happens now? This chapter reviews discharge procedures and options for early discharge.

Early Discharge and Home Care

Managed care, the drive to cut costs, and improved and less invasive medical technologies (such as fiber-optic surgery) have dramatically decreased hospital utilization in the last decade. This book advocates that patients be discharged from the hospital as early as possible, with home care (see Chapter 1) and close outpatient follow-up in the doctor's office to assure ongoing recovery. "Sub-acute" institutions such as *skilled nursing facilities* (nursing homes) are also an option for early discharge. Good candidates for early discharge are described in the following sections.

Infections Treated with Intravenous Antibiotics

If you are admitted to the hospital with an infection requiring five days or a week of IV antibiotics, home care, while an option, offers little benefit over finishing therapy in the hospital. If treatment is going to last weeks to months, as with indolent and hard to treat infections such as *endocarditis* (heart valve infection) or *osteomyelitis* (bone infection), a better plan would be to ask your doctor to arrange home IV infusion. You will need a semi-permanent IV line such as a PICC (see Chapters 1 and 17), training in care of your IV, and training in self-administration of IV antibiotics, but the benefits of being at home to complete treatment—from the security and comfort of a familiar environment to the avoidance of hospital-acquired infections (see Chapter 17)—are obvious.

If you are receiving potentially toxic antibiotics such as an *aminoglycoside* or *vancomycin* (see Chapter 11), a technician will have to come to your house to take periodic blood tests to assure that the levels in your blood are correct—and then report these levels to your doctor—and home health care will give you the means to do so (see Chapter 1).

If you are unable to manage any tasks required of you at home (for example, you are receiving antibiotics too frequently to make home administration practical), your treatment might instead be completed in a skilled nursing facility. Alternatively, ask your doctor about completing treatment with *oral* antibiotics and reporting back to the hospital if you appear to be having a relapse.

Post-Operative Care

As mentioned in Chapter 12, home post-operative care is associated with fewer complications and more rapid recovery than care in the hospital. At the same time, you must be *ready* to go home to avoid rehospitalization. This means your wound should be closed and without signs of infection, all drains must be removed, you must be able to eat (post-operative nausea and vomiting are a common cause of readmission), and your pain must be reasonably well controlled with oral pain medications.

You will need wound care supplies at home, periodic visits by a nurse to check that you are healing properly, follow-up with your surgeon (to remove staples, if any), an ample supply of pain medications, and stool softeners and laxatives to prevent constipation and straining that might cause the wound to reopen.

Physical Rehabilitation

People who are disabled by a stroke might need physical rehabilitation to relearn the skills necessary to function at home (for example, using a walker or cane, or transferring from a wheel-chair to a bed or toilet). Patients might also need physical rehabil-itation after prolonged bed rest. Both tasks can be accomplished with home visits by a physical therapist or, if you are completely unable to care for yourself, in a skilled nursing facility.

Remember that most insurance plans as well as Medicare will provide a home attendant or a home health aide to assist you with light household chores (for example, cooking, shopping, and laundry) and personal care (bathing and dressing), so long as you also have a skilled nursing need. Both services will lapse when your skilled nursing need comes to an end.

Treatment with Blood Thinners

Blood clots (for example, *deep venous thrombosis,* DVT—see Chapter 17) are treated with blood thinners (*anticoagulants*). Traditionally, this has meant admission to the hospital for IV heparin infusion (followed by oral doses of warfarin [Couma-din]), with frequent blood tests to monitor anticoagulation and prevent bleeding. Low-molecular-weight heparin, a new agent (Lovenox, Fragmin), allows treatment to be conducted at home with twice daily injections, without the need for blood tests and a much lower risk of bleeding (see Chapter 11).

Alcohol and Drug Rehabilitation

Alcohol and drug dependence merits a brief period of detox in the hospital followed by transferal to inpatient rehabilitation. Although many alcohol- and drug-addicted patients elect outpa-tient rehab, inpatient treatment offers the best chance for long-term sobriety.

Routine Discharge

Although planning an early discharge is an option for many pa-tients, most will be discharged when the need for acute, hospital-based care is no longer necessary. Many states require 24-hour advance discharge notice to allow patients to prepare for going home. Despite this requirement, discharge can come quite sud-denly (for example, that test you've been waiting for finally happens, and the results are negative); so make sure to communicate with your doctor about when you will be ready.

You should be provided with any prescriptions you need and a follow-up appointment with your doctor. If you have questions about your medications or symptoms that merit closer follow-up, ask them *before* you are discharged. Your nurse or the hospital pharmacist may have pre-printed information on your medications, as well as tasks you will need to perform such as wound care or self administration of insulin, so make sure to ask for this information before you leave.

Medications tend to mount up in the hospital, especially when one or more specialists are involved in your care, and many of them might no longer be needed when you go home. If you are discharged with a fistful of prescriptions, make sure to talk with your doctor about whether all of them are necessary.

Following are some good questions and suggestions for your doctor concerning *hospital discharge:*

- When will I be well enough to go home? Will my therapy last a specific amount of time? What is the end-point?
- Please notify me 24 hours in advance of my discharge.
- Will I be provided with my prescription medications before my discharge, or will I have to fill them? If I do, please provide them to me in advance, so my friend or relative can take them to the pharmacy.
- Can I be discharged early from the hospital and continue my therapy with home care? This is my preference.
- Will I need to continue my recovery (or to recover from my hospitalization) in a skilled nursing facility before I can go home?

Chapter 22

Home Again: Toward a Healthier Tomorrow

So you had a heart attack. You might even have a brand new pacemaker in your chest. You're taking medication for cholesterol and blood pressure, a beta blocker to protect your heart, and an aspirin a day. Now, more than ever, is the time to make sure you take your meds, quit smoking, keep to your diet, and attend regular follow-up exams with your doctor.

Pointers to avoid being rehospitalized include maintaining healthsmart habits by doing the following:

+ Follow a healthy diet and keep your weight down.
+ Don't smoke (or quit smoking).
+ Drink moderately, if at all, and avoid illicit drugs.
+ Practice safe sex.
+ Observe common sense safety precautions such as wearing your seat belt and bicycle helmet.
+ Screen your house for radon.
+ See you doctor regularly for health maintenance.
+ Establish a collaborative relationship with your primary care doctor.
+ Get recommended screening tests (for example, Hepatitis B and C, HIV, pap smear, colonoscopy, and so on).
+ Get recommended vaccinations (flu, pneumovax, hepatitis B, and so on).

- Manage your chronic illness.
- Learn about your illness and participate actively and collaboratively with your doctor in your care.
- Ask *lots* of questions.
- Comply with your regimen of medications.
- Make sure diabetes, hypertension, and other chronic illnesses are well controlled.
- Take HIV medications properly (or not at all).
- Attend regular follow-up exams.

Remember, it is the involved, proactive, and educated patient who is most likely to benefit from a hospital stay and avoid re-admission.

What Does the Future Hold?

What does the future hold for American hospitals and their clients? Heart disease and stroke will continue to be the primary cause of hospitalization and death for the foreseeable future. Although deaths due to cardiovascular disease (CVD) declined 26.1 percent between 1970 and 1980, and 11.4 percent between 1990 and 1997[1], hospitalization for this condition increased by 28 percent from 1979 to 2000, and the aging of the population will lead an increasing *prevalence* (number of existing cases) of *all* chronic disease, including coronary artery disease, heart failure, and stroke[2], as well as hospitalization for these conditions.

Risk factors for CVD will continue to be a problem for millions of Americans. More than 50 percent of Americans are overweight or obese, physical inactivity is increasing, and the decline in adult smoking rates between 1965 and 1995 (from 42 to 25 percent) is now leveling off[1, 3]. The prevalence of diabetes increased by one third between 1990 and 1998[4], and 50 million Americans have high blood pressure, many of whom are either unaware they have the disease or have blood sugar that is poorly controlled[5].

The *incidence* (number of new cases) of cancer increased through the 1970s and 1980s, but leveled off in the 1990s, while cancer mortality rates declined about 1 percent a year from 1993 to 1999. Once again, however, as the population of America ages, the prevalence of cancer will increase, and is expected to double from 1.3 million in 2000 to 2.6 million in 2050[6].

The bottom line? Heart disease will remain the number one killer of Americans and the number one cause of hospitalization for decades to come. Cancer will also cause significant, persisting morbidity and mortality (illness and death). Breakthroughs in the treatment of these illnesses will undoubtedly have positive effects on many millions of people, and mortality rates might continue to decline. Prevention, the most effective long-term management strategy, remains only a partly achieved public health goal.

Cost containment will be the byword of the medical industry for years to come. State and local governments have reached historic levels of debt, with little relief in sight. Medicare and Medicaid, squeezed by these fiscal realities as the number of enrollees reach new highs, will have static and even shrinking budgets. Private insurance and that provided through employee benefit packages will get more expensive, and co-pays for medical services and prescription drugs will increase. The number of uninsured, in the absence of federal and state action, will continue to expand, just as hospitals become less able to provide free care.

A grim picture? Hopefully, by reading the *HealthSmart Hospital Handbook,* you will be able to "hit the ground running" in this newly retrenched health care environment. You're ready to get into the hospital quickly and without the hassle of the emergency room, reduce unnecessary diagnostic procedures, therapies, and medications, and get out as quickly and safely as diligent care allows (to continue therapy at home through home health care, if necessary).

Even better, you, the *potential* patient, will understand the importance of healthy living, regular check-ups and screening with your doctor, and disease management in a collaborative relationship with a primary care physician as a means of avoiding the hospital altogether. By helping you stay *out* of the hospital, the *HealthSmart Hospital Handbook* will have achieved its greatest objective of all.

Glossary

abscess A walled-off collection of pus.

ACE Inhibitors (ACEIs) A class of blood pressure medication.

acetaminophen The active ingredient in Tylenol.

acidosis High acidity of the blood, seen in kidney failure, severe difficulty breathing and other severe medical illness.

activated charcoal An oral slurry of charcoal used in poisonings and overdoses to absorb toxins from the intestines so they do not enter the blood.

activities of daily living (ADLs) Routine daily activities such as eating, dressing, bathing, and using the toilet.

acute Of recent onset (as in *acute illness*).

acute pulmonary edema (APE) Sudden or rapid accumulation of fluid in the lungs, usually resulting from congestive heart failure.

admitting privileges A doctor's ability to admit and care for his or her patients in a hospital.

advanced cardiac life support (ACLS) Chest compressions, ventilation, and the use of medications and electric current to restore electrical activity and a pulse in a patient suffering a *cardiac arrest*.

alcohol withdrawal syndrome (AWS) Tremor, confusion, sweatiness, and other symptoms that follow cessation of alcohol.

alpha blockers A class of blood pressure medication.

allergen A substance or exposure that causes an allergic reaction, such as an insect bite, ragweed, or medication.

ALT (SGPT) A liver enzyme, or transaminase. Elevated in hepatitis and other liver diseases. *See also* liver function tests and SGPT.

altered mental status (AMS) A change in thought patterns or level of consciousness.

alveoli Tiny sacs in the lungs that deliver oxygen into the blood and absorb carbon dioxide.

aminoglycoside   A class of antibiotics that may be especially toxic to the kidneys.

anaphylaxis   A severe allergic reaction, associated with swelling of the face and neck and difficulty breathing.

anasarca   Swelling of the entire body due to extreme excess body fluid.

anemia   Low red blood cells.

angina   Chest pain caused by inadequate blood flow, oxygen, and nutrient delivery to pumping heart muscle.

angiography   Use of contrast dye to outline a blood vessel on x-ray, resulting in an angiogram.

angioplasty   A procedure in which a thin balloon is used to reopen a blocked coronary artery.

antibody   A class of blood proteins (part of the *immune system*) that fight infection and foreign substances and may (in *autoimmune disease*) attack the body's own components.

anticoagulant   A medication that interferes with the ability of the blood to clot (a blood thinner), including heparin and Coumadin (warfarin).

aorta   The main artery of the body, leading from the heart to the chest and abdomen.

aphasia   The inability to speak (or write) coherently (expressive aphasia) or to understand spoken (or written) words (receptive aphasia).

arrhythmia   Abnormal heart rhythm.

arterial blood gas (ABG)   A blood test measuring blood acidity (pH) and oxygen and carbon dioxide levels.

ascites   A collection of fluid in the abdominal cavity, resulting from cirrhosis of the liver, and abdominal cancer and infections.

aspiration   The inhalation of stomach contents and saliva, often resulting in a severe pneumonia.

AST (SGOT)   A *liver enzyme*, or *transaminase*. Elevated in hepatitis and other liver diseases. *See also* liver function tests and SGOT.

asthma   Reversible narrowing of the airways of the lungs, causes periodic bouts of shortness of breath. Often triggered by allergies, air pollution, animal dander, and cigarette smoke.

asymptomatic   Without symptoms.

asystole   Complete cessation of electrical activity of the heart (causing the heart to stop beating).

atherosclerosis   Build-up of fat and other substances in a blood vessel wall, causing narrowing of the blood vessel.

attending   The senior doctor who is medically, ethically, and legally responsible for all aspects of a patient's care.

atrial fibrillation (AF, afib)   An abnormal heart rhythm that is usually rapid and causes irregular pulse.

atypical chest pain   Chest pain that does not fit the usual pattern of pain in a heart attack.

aura   Visual hallucinations, such as sparkling lights or spots, that warn of an impending migraine headache or a seizure. Auras associated with seizures might also be auditory or gustatory.

autoimmune disease   A disease that results from a breakdown in the normal function of the immune system, in which the body's natural defenses against infection attack components of the body itself.

azotemia   An abnormal increase in blood urea nitrogen (BUN) and creatinine in the blood, usually indicating kidney disease.

barium enema   Instillation of a contrast dye into the rectum and large intestine, allowing these structures to be outlined on x-rays.

beta blockers   A class of blood pressure medication.

bicarbonate ($HCO3$, $HCO3-$)   A blood electrolyte, measured in an SMA-7. Important in controlling blood acidity.

bilirubin   A blood pigment that gives stool and urine its color and causes jaundice (icterus). Elevated levels are seen in liver and blood diseases.

biopsy   A small piece of tissue, usually obtained surgically, that is examined in a laboratory to establish a diagnosis.

blood urea nitrogen (BUN)   A nitrogen-containing blood chemical resulting from protein breakdown, used to estimate kidney function and hydration.

board certified   A certification by a nationally recognized authority that minimum requirements for expertise in a given medical or surgical subspecialty, including passing an exam, have been met.

body mass index (BMI)   A measure of weight that takes height into account.

bone scan   A type of nuclear imaging study that shows inflammation in bones, suggestive of cancer, infection, and other bone diseases.

bradycardia   Slow heart beat (fewer than 60 beats per minute).

bright red blood per rectum (BRBPR)   Rectal bleeding.

bronchi (singular: bronchus)   Airways of the lungs.

bronchitis   Inflammation of the airways of the lungs, causing cough, usually due to smoking or a viral illness.

bronchodilator   A class of medicines that cause the airways in the lungs (bronchi) to relax and expand, useful in asthma and COPD.

bronchoscopy   Use of a fiber-optic scope to explore the lungs as an aid in diagnosing severe pneumonia and other lung conditions.

bupropion (Wellbutrin, Zyban)   An antidepressant that is also used to help smoking cessation.

cachexia   Extreme weight loss and wasting due to medical or psychiatric illness.

calcium channel blocker (CCB)   A class of heart and blood pressure medications.

cardiac arrest   Complete cessation of the heart.

cardiac enzymes   Blood chemicals (CPK and troponin) that are elevated in heart attack (myocardial infarction, MI).

cardiologist   Heart specialist.

cardiopulmonary resuscitation (CPR)   Chest compressions and ventilations to maintain blood flow and deliver oxygen to a cardiac arrest victim.

cardiovascular disease (CVD)   A disease of the heart or blood vessels. The most common cause of hospital admission in America.

cardioversion   The use of medications or electric current to convert an abnormal heart rhythm (arrhythmia) to a normal heart rhythm.

CAT scan   *See* CT scan.

cellulitis   Infection of the skin.

cerebrospinal fluid (CSF)   Fluid that bathes the brain and spine. *See also* lumbar puncture.

cervicitis   Inflammation of the cervix, usually due to bacterial (often sexually transmitted) infection.

central line (central venous catheter)   An intravenous catheter placed in a large vein of the neck or chest. A central line may also be threaded from the upper thigh into the abdominal portion of the vena cava.

centrally acting agent   A class of blood pressure medication.

cirrhosis   Scarring and malfunction of the liver.

chest cavity   *See* pleural space.

chest tap   *See* thoracentesis.

chest tube   A plastic tube surgically inserted between two ribs to reinflate a collapsed lung or drain fluid from the chest cavity.

chlamydia   A microorganism that causes sexually transmitted diseases including pelvic inflammatory disease (PID), urethritis, and cervicitis. May also cause newborn pneumonia and eye infections.

chloride (Cl, Cl-)   A blood electrolyte, measured in an SMA-7.

cholelithiasis (gallstones)   Stones in the gall bladder.

chronic bronchitis   Chronic inflammation and narrowing of the airways of the lungs, resulting in wheezing, cough, and shortness of breath. Common in smokers. *See also* chronic obstructive pulmonary disease.

chronic obstructive pulmonary disease (COPD)   A group of chronic lung diseases, including emphysema and chronic bronchitis, characterized by chronic wheezing, cough, and shortness of breath. Common in smokers.

cirrhosis   Severe, end-stage liver disease characterized by scarring of the liver. May lead to ascites, gastrointestinal bleeding, blood coagulation abnormalities, and confusion. Usually caused by alcohol abuse or chronic hepatitis.

Cl (Cl-)   Chloride, a blood electrolyte, measured in an SMA-7.

clostridium difficile (c-diff)   A bacterial infection of the intestines, caused by prolonged antibiotic, that causes severe diarrhea.

coagulation profile   Tests of the blood's clotting ability. Also called PT (prothrombin time) and PTT (partial thromboplastin time).

colon   The large intestine, comprised by the ascending, transverse, and descending colon.

colostomy   A surgical connection between the large intestine (colon) and the skin.

colonoscopy   The use of a fiber-optic scope to look into the colon.

coma (comatose)   Deep unconsciousness. Comatose patients cannot be awakened by light, sound, touch, or pain.

co-morbid   The co-existence of two or more medical conditions in the same patient.

complete blood count (CBC)   A blood test that measures the number, size, and shape of red blood cells, the number and type of white blood cells, and the number of platelets.

concussion   Any violent blow. Usually refers to a traumatic brain injury causing unconsciousness.

conjunctiva   A thin layer of tissue covering the eye and lining the eyelids.

conjunctivitis   Inflammation of the covering of the eye.

congestive heart failure (CHF)   Deterioration in the heart's pumping action, leading to back up of fluid in the lungs.

contractures   Rigid, flexed limbs that follow paralysis in the absence of regular stretching.

contraindication   A circumstance that will cause harm if a specific medication is given (for example, beta blocker medications are contraindicated in asthma).

contrast (contrast dye)   Liquid media that is given by mouth or IV to improve x-ray images.

coronary artery   An artery that supplies the muscle of the heart with oxygenated and nutrient-filled blood.

coronary artery bypass graft (CABG, cabbage [slang])   An operation in which veins are grafted to the coronary arteries to bypass blockages and restore circulation to heart muscle.

coronary heart disease   Heart disease resulting from narrowing and blockage of coronary arteries, including angina and heart attack (myocardial infarction).

corticosteroid (steroid)   A powerful anti-inflammatory drug (including prednisone, Medrol, and others).

costochondritis   Inflammation of the ribs, cartilage, or muscles of the rib cage, a common cause of noncardiac chest pain.

Coumadin (warfarin)   An oral blood thinner (anticoagulant).

CPK   A cardiac enzyme, or blood chemical that is elevated in heart attack. Also called creatine phosphokinase or CK (creatine kinase).

CPR   *See* cardiopulmonary resuscitation.

creatinine   A blood test used to evaluate kidney function, also may be measured in urine.

CT scan   Computed axial tomography (also CAT scan), a special-ized x-ray that shows cross-sectional images of the body.

cystitis   Bladder inflammation.

cystostomy   A surgically created opening between the bladder and the skin.

Darvocet   An oral painkiller combining acetaminophen (Tylenol) and the opiate propoxyphene.

debridement   Cutting away dead and infected tissue from a wound.

deconditioning   Loss of muscle strength and tone, often from pro-longed in-hospital bed rest. Deconditioning happens very rapidly in the elderly, rendering elders unable to get out of bed.

decubitus ulcers   Bedsores.

deep venous thrombosis (DVT)   A blood clot in a major vein.

defibrillation   Use of electric current to convert an abnormal heart rhythm (ventricular fibrillation) to a normal heart rhythm.

delirium tremens (DTs)   Severe shaking, confusion, and hallucina-tions resulting from alcohol cessation.

dementia   A mental condition characterized by impaired memory and intellectual function, and emotional liability.

diabetic ketoacidosis (DKA)   A diabetic condition characterized by very high blood sugar. The high content of glucose in the blood pulls water out of the body, so the patient also becomes dehydrated. DKA is a life-threatening condition.

dialysis   Removal of wastes and toxins from the blood in people with kidney (renal) failure. Includes hemodialysis, which directly "cleans" blood in a dialysis machine, and peritoneal dialysis (which can be done at home), in which fluid is instilled into the abdomen via a catheter and then drained back out.

diplomate   A doctor who has met the requirements for board certi-fication in a medical or surgical specialty area.

defibrillator   An external or internal electric device that treats abnormal heart rhythms. *See also* implanted defibrillator.

disimpaction   Manual removal (with a gloved finger) of stool from the rectum in people unable to move their bowels.

disseminated intravascular coagulation   A blood clotting abnor-mality causing bleeding and clotting throughout the body. Can be fatal.

diuretic   A class of medications that cause urination. Often used to treat high blood pressure and congestive heart failure. Popularly known as water pills.

diverticula (diverticulosis)   Small, baglike pouches in the wall of the large intestine common in the elderly. When infected, a cause of abdominal pain and fever called diverticulitis.

duodenal ulcer (DU)   An erosion in part of the small intestine called the duodenum. Ulcers can cause pain and might bleed or perforate.

duodenum   The part of the small intestine adjacent the stomach.

dyspnea   Shortness of breath.

echocardiogram (echo)   A painless and harmless test that uses sound waves to analyze the structure and function of the heart.

edema   Swelling due to fluid collection in tissue.

effusion   A collection of fluid in a confined space such as the lining of the lungs (pleural effusion) or lining of the heart (pericardial effusion).

elective surgery   A scheduled surgery, such as plastic surgery. Usually not urgent or needed on an imminently life-saving basis.

electrocardiogram (EKG, ECG)   A tracing on paper of the heart's electrical activity. An EKG can help a doctor determine if a patient is having a heart attack, or better, define an abnormal heart rhythm.

electroencephalogram (EEG)   A brain wave test, often done to test for epilepsy (seizure disorder).

embolus (plural: emboli)   A blood clot that breaks off from one area and travels through a blood vessel to become lodged in another area (for example, cerebral embolus).

emesis   Vomiting.

emetic   An agent that induces vomiting.

emphysema   A chronic lung condition in which the airways and air sacs (alveoli) are enlarged and stiffened, causing shortness of breath, cough, and wheezing.

encephalitis   Inflammation of the brain. Can cause temporary coma, and is usually due to viral illness.

endocarditis   An infection of the valves of the heart.

endogastroduodenoscopy (EGD)   The use of a fiber-optic scope to look into the esophagus, stomach, and small intestine.

endoscope   A fiber-optic scope used to see inside the stomach and intestines.

endoscopic retrograde cholangiopancreatography (ERCP)   The use of a fiber-optic scope to look at the pancreatic duct and bile duct.

endotracheal tube   A tube inserted through the mouth into the windpipe (trachea), usually connected to a respirator (ventilator) in people who are unable to breath unassisted.

end-stage disease   The complete failure of an organ system, such as the heart, liver, or kidneys.

epidural   The area adjacent the covering of the spine, often the target of injected anesthesia.

epilepsy   *See* seizure disorder.

epipen   A pre-packaged injectable preparation of epinephrine used to treat severe allergic reactions.

esophageal varices   Engorged veins in the lower part of the esophagus, prone to bleeding. Found in people with cirrhosis, especially in alcoholism and chronic hepatitis. Can cause significant or fatal gastrointestinal bleeding.

esophagus   The swallowing tube, leading from the mouth to the stomach.

essential hypertension   The most common type of high blood pressure, for which no specific cause can be found.

euglycemia   Normal blood sugar (glucose), ranging from 80 to 110 milligrams per deciliter.

expressive aphasia   *See* aphasia.

false negative   A test result suggesting a disease or condition is absent when the disease or condition is present.

false positive   A test result suggesting a disease or condition exists when the disease or condition is absent.

febrile   Having a fever.

fellow   A doctor who has completed a residency program and is continuing to train in a subspecialty area.

fiber optics   A technology that allows internal structures to be seen through a thin, flexible scope.

fibromyalgia   A syndrome, more common in middle-aged women, that causes fatigue and body pain.

fine needle biopsy (or aspiration)   The use of a long, thin needle to take a specimen (biopsy) or a mass or liquid filled space in the body.

fistula   An abnormal (or pathologic) passage between one body cavity and another, or one body cavity and the skin (for example, a rectovaginal fistula connects the rectum and vagina)

focal neurologic deficit (focality)   An abnormality of the function of nerves that indicates damage to the brain or spinal cord. One-sided weakness and unequal pupil size are examples of focal neurologic deficits.

folic acid (folate)   A vitamin necessary for red blood cell production. Folic acid deficiency can cause anemia.

gadolinium   A contrast dye used to improve the cross-sectional images of the body in MRI scans. Rarely causes allergy or kidney damage.

gallstones   *See* cholelithiasis.

gallium scan   A type of nuclear medicine scan that looks for areas of inflammation in the body, possibly due to infection or cancer.

gastric ulcer   An ulcer in the stomach.

gastritis   Inflammation of the stomach, caused by excess acid or infection with *Helicobacter Pylori.*

gastroenteritis (acute gastroenteritis, AGE)   A brief episode of pain and abdominal cramping, often accompanied by nausea, vomiting, and diarrhea. Often viral in origin and popularly called stomach flu.

gastro-esophageal reflux disease (GERD)   Backing up of stomach acid into the esophagus causing chest pain, especially after eating. Popularly know as heartburn.

gastrointestinal (GI) bleeding   Bleeding in the stomach, or small or large intestine.

gastrointestinal system   The organs of digestion, including the mouth, esophagus, stomach, small and large intestine, liver, gall bladder, and pancreas.

GI   Pertaining to the gastrointestinal system.

glucometer   A small, handheld device that measures blood glucose with a single drop of blood. Helps diabetics monitor blood sugar at home.

gout   A form of arthritis that often affects the big toe.

HCO3 (HCO3-) Bicarbonate, a blood electrolyte, measured in an SMA-7. Important in controlling blood acidity.

HDL cholesterol (high density lipoprotein cholesterol) The "good" cholesterol, felt to protect from heart disease.

health-care proxy An individual legally enjoined by a second individual to make medical decisions for the second individual should he or she become unable to advocate for him- or herself. Requires completion of a health-care proxy form.

Helicobacter pylori (*H. Pylori*) A bacteria that causes gastritis and stomach ulcers.

hematemesis Vomiting blood.

hematocrit The percentage of blood comprised by red blood cells, normally 40 to 45 percent.

hematologist A specialist in blood diseases.

hemodialysis *See* dialysis.

hemoglobin A protein that carries oxygen in red blood cells, and gives red cells their color.

hemoglobin A1C A blood test measuring the adequacy of blood glucose control over a period of two to three months, used in diabetes.

hemolysis The breakdown of red blood cells, sometimes causing jaundice (icterus).

hemothorax Blood in the chest cavity.

heparin An injected blood thinner (anticoagulant). May be given by injection to prevent blood clots in bed bound and post-operative patients. *See also* low molecular weight heparin and unfractionated heparin.

hepatitis Inflammation of the liver, usually due to alcohol or a viral infection.

hepatitis A, B, C Inflammation of the liver due to hepatitis A, B, or C virus.

herniated disc Protrusion of the rubbery pad (disc) between two vertebra, causing compression of a nerve and pain in the back and buttock or radiating down one leg.

herpes simplex The cause of cold sores (herpes simplex type I) and genital herpes (herpes simplex type II).

herpes zoster Shingles.

Hickman A type of long term, indwelling central venous catheter. *See also* central line.

HIDA scan A type of nuclear medicine scan that looks for blockages in the liver and bile ducts, possibly due to gallstones.

HIV *See* Human Immunodeficiency Virus.

home attendant Home attendants are licensed by the state and assist patients at home with cooking, shopping, cleaning, and laundry, accompany their charges to doctor's appointments, and might assist with personal care such as feeding and bathing. Home attendants may not administer medications.

home health aide Home health aides are licensed by the state and assist patients at home with personal care such as bathing, feeding, and diaper changing. Home health aides are more trained than home attendants, but also may not administer medications.

hospitalist A doctor specializing in the care of hospitalized patients.

house staff The interns and residents (doctors-in-training) who staff a teaching hospital.

H. Pylori *See Helicobacter pylori.*

Human Immunodeficiency Virus (HIV) The cause of AIDS.

human papilloma virus (HPV) A sexually transmitted viral infection that causes genital warts and can cause cervical cancer.

hyperglycemia Elevated blood glucose (blood sugar), greater than 110 to 120.

hypertension (HTN) Elevated blood pressure, greater than 120 to 130/85 to 90.

hypercholesterolemia Elevated blood cholesterol.

hypoglycemia Low blood sugar, less than 50 to 60.

iatrogenic Illness or injury caused by doctors.

ibuprofen An extremely common over-the-counter painkiller in the nonsteroidal anti-inflammatory agent class of medications (NSAIDs), found in Motrin and Advil.

icterus *See* jaundice.

ideation Thoughts (as in suicidal or homicidal ideation).

ileum Part of the small intestine, adjacent the appendix.

immune system The body's means of protecting itself against infection, including antibodies and white blood cells. May also attack the body's own components, causing *autoimmune disease.*

immunosuppressive An agent or drug that suppresses the immune system, making people more susceptible to infection. Often used to prevent rejection in people who have received organ transplants.

implanted defibrillator A device implanted under the skin of the chest that automatically converts abnormal heart rhythms (arrhythmias) into normal rhythms. May include a pacemaker, which controls heart rate.

incidence The number of new cases of an illness or condition in a given period of time.

infiltrate A hazy area in an x-ray of the lungs, suggestive of pneumonia.

insulin An injected protein used to lower blood sugar in diabetes. *See* lente, regular, and NPH insulin.

intensivist A specialist in critical care such as a cardiologist or pulmonologist who works in an Intensive Care Unit (ICU).

international normalized ratio (INR) A standarized measurement of blood thinning (anticoagulation) used to monitor therapy with Coumadin (warfarin).

intravenous The venous blood stream as a means of administering medications or fluids.

intravenous line (slang: IV) A plastic catheter inserted into a vein as a means of administering medications and fluids.

intravenous pyelogram (IVP) X-rays taken after the administration of intravenous contrast dye that outline the kidneys, ureters, bladder, and urethra. Often used to diagnose kidney stones and blockage of urine flow.

intubation Placing a plastic tube (endotracheal tube) through the mouth and into the windpipe (trachea) and anchoring it in place in order to connect a patient to a respirator (ventilator).

Ipecac *See* Syrup of Ipecac.

isoniazid A medication used in combination with other medications to treat tuberculosis, or as a single agent to treat a positive tuberculosis skin test (PPD, Mantoux test).

IV *See* intravenous and intravenous line.

jaundice (icterus) Yellow-hued skin and eyes resulting from elevated bilirubin in liver disease (and blood diseases causing the breakdown of red blood cells [hemolysis]).

jejenum   Part of the small intestine.

K (K+)   Potassium, a blood electrolyte, measured in an SMA-7.

KUB   An x-ray of the abdomen.

lactated Ringer's (lactated Ringer's solution)   A type of intra-venous fluid preferred by surgeons. Used to hydrate patients who are unable to eat before and after surgery.

lancinating   Lightninglike, or stabbing, as in lancinating pain.

laparoscope   A fiber-optic scope that allows visualization of the abdominal organs through a small incision.

LDL cholesterol (low-density lipoprotein cholesterol)   The bad cholesterol, felt to promote heart disease.

lente insulin   A type of insulin that causes peak blood glucose lowering seven to fifteen hours after administration.

lethargic   Sleepy, but easily arousable.

leukocytis   An elevated white blood cell count, suggestive of an infection.

licensed practical nurse (LPN)   A nurse with lesser training than a registered nurse who might provide some nursing services but may not independently assess or treat patients, and must work under the supervision of an R.N. or M.D.

lidocaine   An anesthetic agent, usually injected to numb a small area.

liver enzyme   *See* transaminase and liver function tests.

liver function tests (LFTs)   A battery of blood tests that measure the health and function of the liver, including the liver enzymes (transaminases, SGOT, also called AST, and SGPT, also called ALT), bilirubin, and alkaline phosphatase.

long-term care   Services that assist people with health or personal needs over a prolonged period of time. Long-term care can be provided at home, or in nursing homes and assisted living facilities. Most long-term care is custodial, rather than skilled nursing, care.

long-term care facility   A residential facility (including assisted living facilities), usually occupied by elderly people, that provides meals, housekeeping services, and personal care services. Most long term care facilities do not provide skilled nursing services (for example, physical therapy or wound care).

loss of consciousness (LOC)   Fainting.

low molecular weight heparin A newer form of the anticoagulant (blood thinner) heparin, given by injection, that is less likely to cause bleeding than unfractionated heparin. Also given to prevent blood clots in bed bound and post-operative patients. Brand names: Fragmin, Lovenox. *See also* heparin and unfractionated heparin.

lower GI (gastrointestinal) bleeding Bleeding from the lower small intestine and large intestine. May cause bloody bowel movements (bright red blood per rectum, BRBPR).

LPN *See* licensed practical nurse.

lumbar puncture (LP) The insertion of a needle into the base of the spine to remove cerebrospinal fluid. Popularly known as a spinal tap.

magnetic resonance imaging (MRI) An imaging technique that uses magnets to create high-resolution cross-sectional images of the body.

mammogram An x-ray screening test for breast cancer.

Mantoux A screening test for tuberculosis. It is not an effective screening test for those who have received BCG. *See* purified protein derivative.

melena Purplish-black, foul smelling feces that result from gastrointestinal bleeding.

meningitis An infection of the covering of the brain and spinal cord.

metastasis (slang: met) A malignant tumor that has spread from a tumor in another area of the body.

metered dose inhaler A handheld device that delivers medication in spray form to be inhaled into the lungs. Popularly known as a pump.

MMR Measles, mumps, and rubella vaccine.

morbidity Sickness.

motor function (motor skills) Voluntary muscle function.

motor vehicle accident (MVA) Car crash.

MRCP An MRI of the gallbladder and bile ducts.

MRI *See* magnetic resonance imaging.

Mycobacterium tuberculosis (MTB) The microorganism that causes tuberculosis.

myocardial infarction (MI) Heart attack.

Na (Na+) Sodium, a blood electrolyte, measured in an SMA-7.

Naproxyn   A common nonsteroidal anti-inflammatory agent (NSAID), and the main ingredient in Naprosyn and Aleve.

nasogastric tube (NG tube)   A plastic catheter inserted through the nose and passed into the stomach.

necrotic   Dead tissue.

needle biopsy   A piece of tissue that is obtained with a needle.

neonatal intensive care unit (NICU)   An intensive care unit for newborns.

nephrolithiasis   Kidney stones.

nephrostomy   A surgically created opening between a kidney and the skin.

nephrotoxin   A medication, poison, or other substance that damages the kidney.

neurologic deficit   *See* focal neurologic deficit.

neuropathy   Dysfunction of a nerve, often resulting in pain or numbness in the hands or feet.

nitrates   A class of heart medication.

nitroglycerine (NTG)   An antianginal medication, often taken under the tongue.

nonketotic hyperosmolar coma (hyperosmolar coma, HOC)   A potentially lethal complication of diabetes characterized by very high blood glucose (blood sugar).

nonsteroidal anti-inflammatory agent (NSAID)   A common class of prescription and nonprescription (over-the-counter) pain relievers, including acetaminophen (Tylenol), ibuprofen (Motrin, Advil) and naproxyn (Naprosyn, Aleve).

nosocomial   Hospital acquired, as in nosocomial infection.

NPH insulin   A type of insulin that causes peak blood glucose lowering four to twelve hours after administration.

NPO   Not allowed to eat.

nuclear medicine (nuclear imaging)   An imaging technology that uses very small doses of radioactive substances to make images of the body that assist in identifying illness.

nurse practitioner   A registered nurse with a master's degree in nursing may assess and treat patients and write prescriptions under the supervision of an M.D.

nurse specialist   A registered nurse who has received additional training in a subspecialty area such as diabetes or AIDS, with a nursing practice focused in this area.

nursing home   *See* skilled nursing facility.

obese   Overweight, with a body mass index of 30 or more.

obstruction   A blockage, usually of the stomach, intestines, or urinary tract, preventing normal movement or food through the digestive system or passage of urine, which may require emergency surgery for relief.

obtunded   A profound decrease in level of consciousness, requiring constant stimulus (for example, shaking) to maintain wakefulness.

occupational therapist   A state licensed specialist in the recovery of functions such as bathing, dressing, and eating lost as a result of hospitalization or illness.

opiate   A class of narcotics with potent pain-killing properties.

orthopnea   Shortness of breath in a recumbent position.

osteoarthritis   The most common form of arthritis, caused by wear and tear on the joints.

osteomyelitis   Bone infection.

osteoporosis   Thin, brittle bones that are easily fractured.

ostomy   A surgically created opening between a hollow organ and the skin (for example, a colostomy is an opening between the colon and the skin). Also called a *stoma*.

pacemaker   A device, usually implanted under the skin (but which may be external on a temporary basis), that uses fine wires and low voltage current to control heartbeat. Often used in people with abnormal or very slow heart rhythms.

pallor   Paleness.

palpitation   A sensation of pounding or a rapid heartbeat in the chest.

pancreatitis   Inflammation of the pancreas, often caused by excessive alcohol intake.

Pap smear   A screening test for cervical cancer.

paracentesis   Inserting a needle into the abdominal cavity to remove fluid (usually ascites).

parenteral   By some means other than through the gastrointestinal tract, usually through the skin. *See also* parenteral nutrition.

parenteral nutrition   Calories, fluids, and nutrients delivered intravenously.

paroxysmal nocturnal dyspnea (PND)   Sudden, severe shortness of breath causing awakening from sleep.

partial thromboplastin time (PTT)   A test of blood clotting, frequently measured in people on intravenous heparin to assure blood is neither over- nor underthinned (anticoagulated).

PE   *See* pulmonary embolism. Also an abbreviation for physical examination.

peak flow   The maximum amount of air that can be exhaled forcefully, measured by a peak flow meter. Useful in assessing the severity of asthma and COPD.

pedal edema   Swelling of the feet and ankles.

pelvic inflammatory disease (PID)   Inflammation of the uterus and fallopian tubes, usually caused by sexually transmitted organisms including gonorrhea and chlamydia.

percutaneous gastrostomy tube (PEG, PEG tube)   A plastic or rubber tube that passes through the abdominal wall into the stomach. Used to feed people who are unable to swallow.

perforation   A hole, usually in the intestine or other hollow organ.

pericardium   A layer of tissue covering the heart.

pH   Acidity, usually of blood. High acidity is seen in severe difficulty breathing and very severe illness.

phlebitis   Inflammation of a vein.

phlebotomy   Blood drawing.

phlebotomist   Blood drawer.

physical therapist   A state licensed specialist in the recovery of physical function such as standing and walking that has been lost after prolonged immobilization or illness.

physician assistant (PA)   A health professional licensed to practice medicine under the supervision of a physician.

PICC line (peripherally inserted central catheter)   A catheter that is inserted into the arm and threaded into the superior vena cava.

platelets   Blood cells that help blood to clot.

pleura   A thin layer of tissue that lines the lungs and chest cavity.

pleural space   The space between the lungs and chest wall, lined by pleura, and usually occupied by the lungs. Also called the chest cavity. May be occupied by air in lung collapse (pneumothorax), blood (hemothorax), or fluid (pleural effusion).

pneumothorax   Air in the pleural space (chest cavity), usually caused by the collapse of a lung.

PO   Taken by mouth, as in medication or fluids and food.

portacath   A type of long-term, indwelling central venous catheter. *See also* central line.

potassium (K, K+)   A blood electrolyte, measured in an SMA-7.

prevalence   The number of cases of an illness or condition in existence at any given time.

primary care   Basic health maintenance and disease management (as in primary care practitioner).

prostate specific antigen   A blood screening test for prostate cancer.

prothrombin time (PT)   A test of blood clotting, measured weekly or more often in people taking Coumadin (warfarin) to assure blood is neither over- nor underthinned (anticoagulated).

pulmonary edema   *See* acute pulmonary edema.

pulmonary embolism (PE)   A blood clot in the lungs.

pulmonary function tests   Measurements of air flow rates in the lung and lung volume, useful in assessing the severity of asthma and COPD and the response of these illnesses to medications.

pulmonologist   A doctor who specializes in the treatment of lung diseases.

pump   *See* metered dose inhaler.

purified protein derivative (PPD, Mantoux)   A skin test for infection with Mycobacterium tuberculosis (MTB), the cause of tuberculosis. A positive test indicates only the presence of MTB, not active disease.

pyelonephritis   Kidney infection.

QID   Four times a day.

radiograph   X-ray.

rales   A fine crackling sound heard in the lungs, especially in pneumonia.

red blood cell (RBC)   Oxygen carrying blood cell that gives blood its color.

registered nurse (RN)   A nurse with an associate or baccalaureate degree, licensed by a state to practice nursing. May independently assess and treat patients.

regular insulin   A type of insulin that causes peak blood glucose lowering two and a half to five hours after administration.

renal   Having to do with the kidneys.

renal failure   Kidney failure, usually necessitating dialysis. Urine may continue to be produced in some forms of renal failure.

renal insufficiency   Malfunctioning kidneys, usually not requiring dialysis. Urine continues to be produced.

resident   A doctor in training who has already completed the internship year.

respiratory therapist   A state licensed technician with an associate or baccalaureate degree who administers inhaled medications, operates respirators, and performs other functions related to the diagnosis and treatment of lung diseases.

RN   *See* registered nurse.

RPR   A newer form of blood testing for syphilis. Also called rapid plasma reagin.

rubella   A viral infection that can cause birth defects, also called German measles.

rule-out myocardial infarction   An admission diagnosis in patients with chest pain who might be having a heart attack. Blood tests to measure cardiac enzymes (CPK and troponin) and electrocardigrams (EKGs) are conducted over 24 hours to establish (rule-in) or exclude (rule-out) heart attack.

saline   A type of intravenous fluid comprised of water and salt, commonly used in hospitals.

seizure   Abnormal electrical activity of the brain, often resulting in loss of consciousness and a convulsion. *See also* tonic-clonic seizure.

seizure disorder   A disease characterized by recurrent seizures. Also called epilepsy.

sepsis   A severe blood infection.

SGOT (AST)   A liver enzyme (transaminase) that can be measured in blood. Elevated levels are found in hepatitis.

SGPT (ALT)   A liver enzyme (transaminase) that can be measured in blood. Elevated levels are found in hepatitis.

shock   A profound, life-threatening reduction in blood pressure.

sigmoid colon   A section of the colon (large intestine) near the rectum and anus.

sigmoidoscopy   The use of a fiber-optic scope to look at the sigmoid colon (large intestine).

singultus   Hiccups.

sinus   A blind opening or space.

skilled nursing facility (SNF)   A healthcare facility specializing in providing skilled nursing care (for example, wound care), physical therapy, and other professional services. Popularly called a nursing home.

sleep apnea   Brief periods of respiratory arrest during sleep, usually accompanied by loud snoring.

SMA-7 (slang: smack)   A battery of blood tests measuring sodium, potassium, chloride, bicarbonate, BUN, creatinine, and glucose.

SOB   Shortness of breath.

sodium (Na, Na+)   A blood electrolyte, measured in an SMA-7.

sodium chloride (NaCl)   Salt. Usually refers to a type of intravenous fluid combining salt and water in common use in hospitals. *See also* saline.

spacer   A clear plastic tube connected to a metered dose inhaler to improve the delivery of inhaled medication to the lung.

statins   A class of cholesterol-lowering medications (also called HMG Co-A reductase inhibitors).

staphylococcus (staphylococcus aureus, staph)   A virulent bacteria that causes serious skin and blood infections, pneumonia, abscesses, and other types of infections.

STD   Sexually transmitted disease.

stenosis   Narrowing of a hollow space or lumen of a tube (for example, stenosis of the bile duct).

steroid   *See* corticosteroid.

stoma   *See* ostomy.

stress test   A test that evaluates the heart for coronary artery disease (narrowing of the coronary arteries).

stricture   A bandlike narrowing of a hollow space or lumen of a tube (for example, an intestinal stricture).

stroke (cerebrovascular accident, CVA)   Death of a portion of the brain, usually due to a narrowed blood vessel or a blood clot, causing neurologic problems such as one-sided weakness, slurred speech, and aphasia.

subcutaneous (sub-Q)   Under the skin (for example, subcutaneous injection).

sudden death   Sudden cessation of the heart and breathing, usually the result of a lethal arrhythmia (abnormal heart rhythm).

supratentoral   (slang) A condition that is imaginary or "in the patient's head."

supraventricular tachycardia (SVT)   A type of arrhythmia characterized by an abnormally rapid heart rate (greater than 150 to 160 beats per minute).

sutures   Stitches.

syphilis   A sexually transmitted infection initially characterized by a painless genital ulcer. May cause neurologic, cardiac, and other problems if untreated after many years.

syncope   Fainting from any of a number of causes.

Syrup of Ipecac   A liquid emetic, used to induce vomiting in overdoses and poisonings.

tachycardia   Heart rate of 100 or more.

tap   (slang) Use a needle to remove fluid (for example, chest tap).

telemetry   Constant monitoring of a patient's heart rhythm and other vital functions.

thoracentesis   Insertion of a needle or catheter to remove fluid from the pleural space (chest cavity). Also called chest tap.

thrombus   Blockage of a blood vessel (plural: thrombi).

TID   Three times a day.

tinnitus   Ringing in the ears.

tonic-clonic seizure   A generalized convulsion with loss of consciousness, incontinence, and often with tongue biting.

trachea   Windpipe.

tracheostomy   A surgically created connection between the trachea (windpipe) and skin.

transaminase   A liver enzyme, SGOT (or AST) or SGPT (or ALT). Elevated levels are seen in hepatitis and other liver disease.

transdermal   Through the skin, especially as a mode of medication delivery (for example, the pain medication fentanyl can be given transdermally with a patch).

triage   Prioritizing newly arrived patients in the emergency room to see a doctor depending on the urgency of their condition.

triglyceride   A type of fat.

troponin   A blood chemical that is elevated in heart attack (myocardial infarction, MI).

ulcers, gastric and duodenal   Gastric ulcers are painful erosions in the wall of the stomach, often caused by excess acid, alcohol, or infection with a bacteria called *Helicobacter pylori* (*H. Pylori*). Duodenal ulcers (DU) are located in the duodenum; the part of the intestine that is right next to the stomach.

unfractionated heparin   An older form of the anticoagulant (blood thinner) heparin, given by intravenous infusion, and more prone to cause bleeding than low molecular weight heparin. May be given by injection to prevent blood clots in bed bound and post-operative patients.

upper gastrointestinal bleeding (upper GI bleeding)   Bleeding from the upper small intestine or stomach, causing vomiting of blood or digested blood (coffee ground emesis).

upper gastrointestinal series (upper GI series)   X-rays taken after drinking contrast dye, outlining the stomach and small intestine.

ureters   Paired tubes that connect the kidneys to the bladder.

urethra   The lower end of the urinary tract, extending from the bladder to the perineum (in women) or the glans penis (in men).

urethritis   Inflammation of the urethra, usually due to bacterial (often sexually transmitted) infection.

urinalysis (U/A)   A battery of urine tests, useful in diagnosing urinary infection, kidney stones, and other conditions of the urinary tract.

urine culture (U/C)   A test for bacteria in urine, useful in diagnosing urinary infection.

Vancomycin   A potent intravenous antibiotic used to treat virulent and resistant bacterial infections.

varicella   A viral infection that causes a bumpy, red, scabbed rash, also called chicken pox.

varices   Blood engorged veins.

vasovagal syncope   A simple faint, also called a common faint, due to emotional distress or other stressors.

vena cava   The main vein of the body, leading to the heart from the abdomen and chest.

ventilator   A machine used to force air (or oxygen) into the lungs in people unable to breathe unassisted. Popularly know as a respirator.

ventricular fibrillation (VF, V-fib)   A chaotic heart rhythm, uniformly fatal if untreated.

ventricular tachycardia (VTach)   A very rapid heart rhythm (arrhythmia), usually fatal if untreated.

viral syndrome   A minor viral illness such as a stomach flu or cold that resolves on its own.

vital signs (vitals)   Blood pressure, pulse, respiratory rate, and temperature.

white blood cell (WBC)   A blood cell that helps protect the body from infection. Measured with a CBC (complete blood count) and elevated in the presence of infection.

zoster   *See* herpes zoster.

Appendix B

Bibliography

Introduction

[1] *National Hospital Discharge Survey, Annual Summary,* Centers for Disease Control and Prevention (CDC), Department of Health and Human Services, 1999.

[2] *Guidelines for the Diagnosis and Management of Asthma,* U.S. Department of Health and Human Services, National Institutes of Health, No. 91-3042, 1991.

Chapter 1

[1] Freeman, Laura. "Home Sweet Home Health Care," *Monthly Labor Review,* March 1995.

Chapter 2

[1] Silverman, E., S. Skinner et al. "The Association Between For-Profit Hospital Ownership and Increased Medicare Spending," *New England Journal of Medicine,* August 5, 1999.

[2] Green, H. R., B. J. Packard et al. "When Money Is the Mission—The High Costs of Investor-Owned Care," *New England Journal of Medicine,* August 5, 1999.

Chapter 3

[1] *To Err Is Human: Building a Safer Health System,* Institute of Medicine, November 1999.

2 "Preventing Medical Errors," *The New York Times*, A-22, December 1, 1999.

3 Weiss, R. "Medical Errors Blamed for Many Deaths—as Many as 98,000 a Year in U.S. Linked to Mistakes," *Washington Post*, November 30, 1999, A-1.

4 "Deaths Due to Medical Error Are Exaggerated in the Institute of Medicine Report," *Journal of the American Medical Association*, 284(1), July 5, 2000.

5 *Managed Care Fact Sheets*, Managed Care National Statistics, Managed Care On-Line (www.mcareol.com).

6 "Managed Care Profits Come from Physician's Pockets," *American Medical News*, September 2, 2002.

7 Toner, R., and S. G. Stolberg. "Decade After Health Care Crisis, Soaring Costs Bring New Strains," *The New York Times*, August 11, 2002.

8 "Medicare Cuts to Slash Patient Care by $2.88 Billion," *Elder Life Planning Café*, March 27, 2002.

9 *Medicare Cuts Physician Payments 28.1 Percent*, U.S. Newswire, American College of Physicians—American Society of Internal Medicine, February 28, 2002.

10 Hawryluk, M. "Doctors Could Face Four Years of Medicare Payment Cuts," *American Medical News*, March 18, 2002.

11 *2000 Annual Report*, National Practitioner Data Bank, 2000.

12 Treaster, J. "Rise in Insurance Forces Hospitals to Shutter Wards," *The New York Times*, August 25, 2002.

13 *Nursing Shortage Poses Serious Health Care Risk: Joint Commission Expert Panel Offers Solutions to National Healthcare Crisis*, Joint Commission on Accreditation of Healthcare Organizations, News Room, News Release Archives, August 7, 2002.

14 *Health Care at the Crossroads: Strategies for Addressing the Evolving Nursing Crisis*, Joint Commission on Accreditation of Healthcare Organizations, August 7, 2002.

15 *Drowning in a Sea of Paperwork*, Pricewaterhouse Coopers/ American Hospital Association, 2002.

Chapter 4

1 Billings, J., and N. Parikh. *Emergency Room Use: The New York Story,* The Commonwealth Fund, October 2000.

2 Billings, J., N. Parikh, and T. Mijanovich. *Emergency Department Use in New York City: A Survey of Bronx Patients,* The Commonwealth Fund, November 2000.

3 Brownfield, E. *Use of Analgesics in the Acute Abdomen,* Agency for Healthcare Research and Quality, www.ahcpr/clinic/ptsafety/cha37a.htm.

4 Lurie, P. *Statement on Safety Issues Related to Acetaminophen Before the Nonprescription Drugs Advisory Committee* (HRG Publication #1639), Public Citizen's Health Research Group, September 19, 2002.

5 Stolberg, S. G. "Warnings Sought for Popular Painkiller," *The New York Times,* September 20, 2002.

6 Ko, C., and F. Tilden. "Toxicity, Nonsteroidal Anti-Inflammatory Agents," *E-medicine,* www.emedicine.com, June 14, 2001.

7 *Preventing Iron Poisoning in Children,* U.S. Food and Drug Administration, FDA Backgrounder, January 15, 1997.

Chapter 5

1 *Conditions of Participation for Hospitals, Code of Federal Regulations,* Title 42, Volume 3, Parts 430 to End, U.S. Government Printing Office, 42CFR482.1, revised as of October 1, 1999.

2 Bottrell, M., and A. Hillel et al. *Hospital Informed Consent for Procedure Forms,* Archives of Surgery, 135:1 (26–33), January 2000.

Chapter 8

1 "Articles Warn Against Phlebotomy Induced Anemia," *Phlebotomy Today,* 2(6), June 2001.

2 *Questions and Answers,* Health Physics Society, www.hps.
org/publicinformation/ate/q420.html, December 1, 2000.
3 *Radiological Preparedness,* Nebraska Emergency
Management Agency, 2002.
4 Fearon, W. "Post-Lumbar Puncture Headache," *P & S
Medical Review,* 1(2), March 1994.
5 Follens, I., and D. Godts et al. "Combined Fourth and Sixth
Cranial Nerve Palsy After Lumbar Puncture: A Rare
Complication. A Case Report." *Bulletin de la Société Belge
d'Ophtalmologie,* 281, 29–33, 2001.

Chapter 10
1 Beers, M., and R. Berkow, ed. *The Merck Manual of
Diagnosis and Therapy, 17th Edition,* 1-1, Nutrition: General
Considerations, 1999.

Chapter 12
1 "Benefits of Ambulatory Surgery," *Miller: Anesthesia, Fifth
Edition,* 65, Churchill Livingston, Inc., 2000.
2 Auerbach, A. D., and L. Goldman. "Beta Blockers and
Reduction of Cardiac Events in Non-Cardiac Surgery,"
Journal of the American Medical Association, 287 (11),
March 20, 2002.
3 Di Nicola, Aniello. *Post-Operative Pain Management, The
Virtual Anesthesia Textbook,* 2000.
4 Newman, M. F., and J. L. Kirchner. "Perioperative Neuro-
cognitive Decline Following CABG's Was Persistent and
Associated with Later Cognitive Decline," *Evidence Based
Cardiovascular Medicine,* 5(2), June 2001.
5 *Infectious Risks of Blood Transfusion,* Blood Developments,
Blood Centers of the Pacific, Publication No. 16., February
2002.
6 *About Risks of Blood Transfusion, Health Care Acquired
Infections Division Transfusion-Transmitted Injuries Section,*
Population and Public Health Branch, Health Canada, June
2002.

[7] Reger, T. B., and D. Roditski. "Bloodless Medicine and Surgery for Patient Having Cardiac Surgery," *Critical Care Nurse,* 21(4), August 2001.

[8] *Regional Anesthesia for Ambulatory Surgery,* Anesthesia Clinics of North America, 18-2, June 2000.

Chapter 13

[1] Justic, M. "Does ICU Psychosis Really Exist?" *Critical Care Nurse,* 20 (3), June 2000.

[2] Teni, J. M., and E. Fisher. "Decision Making and Outcomes of Prolonged ICU Stays in Seriously Ill Patients," *Journal of the American Geriatric Society,* 48(5):S70, May 4, 2000.

Chapter 14

[1] "The SUPPORT Principal Investigators: A Controlled Trial To Improve Care for Seriously Ill Hospitalized Patients: The Study to Understand Prognoses and Preferences for Outcomes and Risks of Treatment (SUPPORT)," *Journal of the American Medical Association,* 274:1591-8, 1995.

[2] *Acute Pain Management, Operative or Medical Procedures and Trauma, Clinical Practice Guideline,* Agency for Heathcare Research and Quality, February 1992.

[3] *The World Health Organization's Three-Step Analgesic Ladder,* World Health Organization, 1990.

[4] White, P. F. "Use of Patient Controlled Analgesia for Management of Acute Pain," *Journal of the American Medical Association,* 259:243, 1988.

[5] "Patient Controlled Analgesia," *Miller: Anesthesia, Fifth Edition,* 2326–2327, 2000.

Chapter 17

[1] *New York State Mandatory Infection Control and Barrier Precautions Course,* 2002.

[2] *Nosocomial Infections in Healthcare Facilities, Risk Management Review,* The Reciprocal Group, March 2001.

[3] *New York State Mandatory Infection Control and Barrier Precautions Course,* 2002.

[4] Bures, S. et al. "Computer Keyboards and Faucet Handles as Reservoirs of Nosocomial Pathogens in the ICU," *American Journal of Infection Control,* 28:465–470, 2000.

[5] Guilhermetti, M., and S. Hernandes et al. "Effectiveness of Hand-Cleansing Agents for Removing Methcillin Resistant Staphylococcus from Contaminated Hands," *Infection Control and Hospital Epidemiology,* 22(1), February 2001.

[6] "Doctors Are Told Alcohol Gels Are Better Than Soap and Water," *The New York Times,* October 26, 2002.

[7] *Nosocomial Infections and Infection Control in the Hospital,* Department of Community and Preventive Medicine, Joseph A. Cimino, M.D., chairman.

[8] O'Grady, N. P., and M. Alexander et al. "Guidelines for the Prevention of Intravascular Catheter Related Infections," *Mor- bidity and Mortality Weekly Report,* 51, RR-10, 9 August 2002.

[9] "The Prevention and Treatment of Pressure Sores," *Effective Health Care,* 2(1), October 1995.

Chapter 18

[1] "Current Trends Hospitalizations for the Leading Causes of Death Among the Elderly—United States," *Morbidity and Mortality Weekly Report,* 39(43); 777–779, 785, November 2, 1990.

[2] Sahyoun, N. R., and H. Lentzner et al. "Trends in Causes of Death Among the Elderly," *Aging Trends,* 1, Hyattsville, Maryland: National Center for Health Statistics, 2001.

[3] Somogyi-Zalud, E. *Hazards of Hospitalization in the Elderly,* Washington VAMC and the George Washington University Medical Center, April 1999.

Chapter 19

[1] Tierney, L., and S. McPhee, ed. "Cirrhosis," *Lange Current Medical Diagnosis and Treatment,* 677–682, 2001.

[2] *NHLBI Funded Study Finds Heart Assist Device Extends and Improves Lives of Patients with End-Stage Heart Failure,* NIH News Release, National Institutes of Health, November 12, 2001.

[3] Christakis, N., and E. Lamont. "Extent and Determinants of Error in Doctors' Prognoses in Terminally Ill Patients: A Prospective Cohort Study." *British Medical Journal,* 320; 7233:469–473.

[4] "The SUPPORT Principle Investigators: A Controlled Trial To Improve Care for Seriously Ill Hospitalized Patients. The Study to Understand Prognoses and Preferences for Outcomes and Risks of Treatment (SUPPORT)," *Journal of the American Medical Association,* 274:1591–8, 1995.

[5] Wilson, I. B. et al. "Is Experience a Good Teacher? How Interns and Attending Physicians Understand Patients' Choices for End-of-Life Care." *Medical Decision Making,* 17(2): 217–27, April–June 1997.

Chapter 22

[1] National Conference on Cardiovascular Disease Prevention: Meeting Healthy People, 2010 Objectives for Cardiovascular Health, Bethesda, MD, 2002.

[2] *Heart Disease and Stroke, 2003 Update,* American Heart Association, 2003.

[3] "Achievements in Public Health, 1900–1999: Decline in Deaths from Heart Disease and Stroke—United States, 1900–1999," *Morbidity and Mortality Weekly Report,* 48(30), 649–656, August 6, 1999.

[4] Mokdad, A. H., and E. S. Ford et al. "Diabetes Trends in the U.S.: 1990–1998," *Diabetes Care,* 23(9), 1278–83, 2000.

[5] *The Sixth Report of the Joint National Committee on Prevention, Detection, Evaluation, and Treatment of High*

Blood Pressure, National Institutes of Health, National Heart, Lung, and Blood Institute, November 1997.

[6] "Annual Report to the Nation on the Status of Cancer, 1973–1999, Featuring Implications of Age and Aging on the U.S. Cancer Burden," *Cancer,* 94(10), 2766–2792, May 15, 2002.

Index

Index